Handbook of

Human Tissue Sources

T0130714

A National Resource of Human Tissue Samples

Elisa Eiseman
Susanne B. Haga

Supported by the
Office of Science and Technology Policy

Science and Technology Policy Institute

RAND

One aspect of the recent and rapid advances in biological and medical research is that human tissue is being used in an increasing variety of new ways. Now that techniques exist to extract DNA from minuscule archival samples, including frozen blood or tissue samples and even paraffin-embedded tissue blocks, genetic tests could potentially be performed on virtually any size stored tissue sample. These technological advances, which have been so instrumental in recent biomedical discoveries, have also raised several legal, ethical, and societal issues, including concerns about privacy and informed consent.

To assist in their examination of the issues associated with the use of stored tissue samples, the National Bioethics Advisory Commission (NBAC) requested information about the magnitude of the existing archives of tissues in the United States from the Science and Technology Policy Institute at RAND. The commissioned report represented the first inventory of stored tissue sample repositories in the United States. The report provided information about major tissue storage facilities and information about several aspects of stored tissue samples, such as how many tissue samples exist in the United States, where they are, who has access to them, and for what purposes they are used. This handbook is an extension of the NBAC-commissioned report and represents a comprehensive inventory of stored human biological materials in the United States. The handbook is the first of its kind and should be extremely useful to scientific researchers throughout the world.

Originally created by Congress in 1991 as the Critical Technologies Institute and renamed in 1998, the Science and Technology Policy Institute is a federally funded research and development center sponsored by the National Science Foundation and managed by RAND. The institute's mission is to help improve public policy by conducting objective, independent research and analysis on policy issues that involve science and technology. To this end, the institute

- Supports the Office of Science and Technology Policy and other Executive Branch agencies, offices, and councils

- Helps science and technology decisionmakers understand the likely consequences of their decisions and choose among alternative policies

- Helps improve understanding in both the public and private sectors of the ways in which science and technology can better serve national objectives.

Science and Technology Policy Institute research focuses on problems of science and technology policy that involve multiple agencies. In carrying out its mission, the institute consults broadly with representatives from private industry, institutions of higher education, and other nonprofit institutions.

Inquiries regarding the Science and Technology Policy Institute or this document may be directed to:

Bruce Don, Ph.D.
Director, Science and Technology Policy Institute
RAND
1333 H Street, N.W.
Washington, D.C. 20005
Phone: (202) 296-5000
Web: http://www.rand.org/centers/stpi/
Email: stpi@rand.org

CONTENTS

Appendix

FIGURES

TABLES

In the United States, human tissues have been stored for more than 100 years. Some institutions in the United States have archived specimens of human tissues that are more than 100 years old. Historically, these stored tissue samples have been used by the biomedical community for educational and research purposes. More recently, stored tissues have played a major role in the understanding and treatment of such diseases as cancer, HIV/AIDS, and heart disease. However, the use and storage of human tissues raises several legal, ethical, and societal issues. Furthermore, as recent and rapid advances in biological and medical research have made it possible to analyze DNA from almost any minuscule sample of human tissue, concerns about privacy and informed consent have been raised. Complicating these issues is the paucity of information addressing tissue acquisition, use, and storage.

To date, no central database captures information about stored tissue samples. Therefore, the National Bioethics Advisory Commission (NBAC) initially requested information about stored tissue samples in the United States for its report on research involving human biological materials to obtain a better understanding of the magnitude of existing archives. This handbook is an extension of that report, and its purpose is to collect for the first time, in a single document, information about tissue storage in the United States. It also provides information about several aspects of stored tissue samples, such as how many tissue samples exist in the United States, where they are, who has access to them, and for what purposes they are used. The completion of this handbook coincides with the recent release of NBAC's final report, "Research Involving Human Biological Materials: Ethical Issues and Policy Guidance." (NABC, 1999.)

A conservative estimate from the tissue collections described in this book is that more than 307 million tissue specimens from more than 178 million cases are stored in the United States, accumulating at a rate of more than 20 million per year. These tissue collections vary considerably, ranging from formal repositories to the informal storage of blood or tissue specimens in a researcher's freezer. Archives of human tissue range in size from fewer than 200 to more than 92 million specimens.

The two largest tissue repositories in the world, the National Pathology Repository and the DNA Specimen Repository for Remains Identification, are housed within a single institution, the Armed Forces Institute of Pathology (AFIP). These two repositories alone store more than 94 million specimens. The tissue repositories supported by the NIH are not as large as those at AFIP, but the NIH is probably the largest funder of extramural tissue repositories, supplying more than $53 million in fiscal year 1996. Finally, the pathology departments at graduate medical education (GME) teaching institutions collectively constitute the largest and oldest stores of tissue samples in the United States with some specimens more than a century old.

The vast majority of tissues were originally collected for diagnostic or therapeutic reasons. Three sources, the AFIP National Pathology Repository, GME teaching institution pathology departments, and newborn screening laboratories, represent more than 265.5 million diagnostic and therapeutic specimens from more than 176 million cases. Tissues collected for diagnostic or therapeutic reasons can sometimes be used for research, educational, and quality-control purposes, but the vast majority are not.

Several repositories have been established specifically for research. In addition, several very large longitudinal studies collect and bank samples from their study participants. Likewise, a fair amount of research simultaneously creates tissue collections or contributes to tissue banks. Collectively, these tissue collections contain more than 2.3 million specimens. Because these tissues are collected specifically for research purposes, it is not surprising that the use of these tissues has resulted in numerous research publications.

Other than for diagnostic and therapeutic purposes or for use in research, tissues are collected and stored for a variety of reasons. Blood banks collect approximately 12 million units of blood a year, but only about 20,000 to 40,000 units are stored at any one time. Also, most of the blood collected is used for transfusions, and very little is used for such other purposes as research and quality control. Organ banks do not collect the same volume of tissue that blood banks do but are very similar in the respect that most of the organs and tissues collected are used for transplants, and very little is available for research. Forensic DNA banks collect and store tissues for use in criminal investigations. The DoD DNA Specimen Repository and some commercial DNA banks store DNA samples for remains identification. Sperm, ovum, and embryo banks store specimens for anonymous donation or for later use by the individual storing the material. Umbilical cord blood banks also store blood for anonymous donation and later use by families banking their newborn's cord blood.

Many valuable specimens and data resources exist from a variety of sources, but no centralized database allows researchers to obtain access to and information about them. This RAND handbook brings together information about several sources of stored tissue samples in the United States. It represents the first time that this information has been assembled in a single publication and the first time the magnitude of the archives of stored tissues has been assessed. This handbook may serve as a reference for researchers to identify potential tissue resources. It may also serve as a basis for developing a national database. This handbook will be a valuable resource for researchers who require tissue samples for studies in genetics, cancer, immunology, physiology, and cell biology, among other disciplines. In addition, this handbook will be useful to policymakers, physicians, and other health-care professionals.

ACKNOWLEDGMENTS

The authors would like to thank several people who contributed to this handbook:

Jennifer Brower from RAND who executed the RaDiUS database searches, contacted references, performed background research, and reviewed the document; Sheri Alpert, a medical privacy expert, for seminal papers on DNA banking, substantive discussions, and critical review; Fran Pitlick from the Federation of American Societies for Experimental Biology who provided invaluable information about stored tissue samples at GME teaching institution pathology laboratories and arranged for the meeting with the chairs of pathology at the Universities Associated for Research and Education in Pathology meeting; Ginny Levin from George Washington University for providing useful information and informed consent forms from the Women's Health Initiative longitudinal study as well as general consent forms for diagnostic and therapeutic obstetrical and gynecological procedures; Jayne Hart Chambers, Kathleen O'Donaghue, and Henry Travers from the College of American Pathologists (CAP), for providing documents about the types of laboratories that CAP accredits and the CAP statement on laboratory regulation to the Task Force on Genetic Testing; Philippe Bishop from the National Cancer Institute (NCI), who engaged in substantive discussions and critically reviewed this document; Tom Moore, the CEO of Cord Blood Registry, for valuable information about umbilical cord blood banking; Sheila Taube and Marianna Bledsoe from the NCI for useful information about NCI-funded tissue banks; Michael Peterson from the Armed Forces Institute of Pathology (AFIP), who supplied detailed information about the AFIP National Pathology Repository; Lynn Agostini, Ianve Clark, and Janice Smith from the American Red Cross, who provided information about American Red Cross blood banking and tissue services; Brett Fritz from the Eastern Cooperative Oncology Group (ECOG), who supplied information about ECOG tissue banking; Gladys White from the National Advisory Board on Ethics in Reproduction (NABER), for information on assisted reproduction technologies and fertility clinics; Capt. William D. Wurzel, a pathologist at the

Bureau of Medicine and Surgery, U.S. Navy, who supplied information and contact names for Navy pathology and blood banking services; Jean McEwen from Boston College School of Law, who suggested people to contact for information on DNA banking; Richard A. Rettig and Thomas L. Lincoln from RAND, for critically reviewing this document; Beth Lachman from RAND, for her mathematical modeling expertise; Donna Fossum and David Trinkle from RAND, for guidance on the use of the RaDiUS database; Dan Sheehan from RAND, for editing the manuscript; Lisa Sheldone from RAND, for her administrative expertise in bringing this project to fruition; Birthe Wenzel from RAND, for her computer expertise; and everyone who provided valuable information about sources of stored tissue samples described in this report.

ABBREVIATIONS

ACTG	AIDS Clinical Trials Group
ADA	American Diabetes Association
AFDIL	Armed Forces DNA Identification Laboratory
AFIP	Armed Forces Institute of Pathology
AIDS	Acquired Immune Deficiency Syndrome
ALL	Acute lymphoblastic leukemia
AMB	AIDS Malignancy Bank
AM-CTC	AIDS-Malignancy Clinical Trials Consortium
AML	Acute myelogenous leukemia
ARC	Alzheimer's Research Center
ARNC	Army-Navy Serum Repository
ART	Assisted reproductive technology
ASCO	American Society of Clinical Oncology
BBDR	Benign Breast Disease Registry
BTR	Breast Tissue Repository
CALGB	Cancer and Leukemia Group B
CAP	College of American Pathologists
CBCTR	Cooperative Breast Cancer Tissue Resource
CCCBB	Chicago Community Cord Blood Bank
CCG	Children's Cancer Group
CCOP	Community Clinical Oncology Program
CDC	Centers for Disease Control and Prevention
cDNA	Complementary DNA (deoxyribonucleic acid)

CFRBCS	Cooperative Family Registry for Breast Cancer Studies
CGOP	Cooperative Group Outreach Program
CHR	Center for Health Research
CHTN	Cooperative Human Tissue Network
CJD	Creutzfeldt-Jakob disease
CLIA	Clinical Laboratory Improvement Amendments
CLSS	Central Laboratory Services Section
CME	Continuing Medical Education
CMV	Cytomegalovirus
CNS	Central nervous system
CNSC	Central Nervous System Consortium
CODIS	Combined DNA Index System
CPP	Collaborative Perinatal Project
CRISP	Computer Retrieval of Information on Scientific Projects
CTI	Critical Technologies Institute
DIEP	Diabetes in Early Pregnancy Study
DISC	Diet Intervention Study in Children
DNA	Deoxyribonucleic acid
DoD	Department of Defense
EBV	Epstein-Barr virus
ECOG	Eastern Cooperative Oncology Group
EPA	Environmental Protection Agency
EST	Expressed Sequence Tag
FASEB	Federation of American Societies for Experimental Biology
FBI	Federal Bureau of Investigation
FDA	Food and Drug Administration
GIVF	Genetics and IVF Institute
GME	Graduate medical education
GOG	Gynecologic Oncology Group
GVHD	Graft versus host disease

H&E	Hematoxylin and Eosin
HBDI	Human Biological Data Interchange
HD	Hodgkin's disease
HHANES	Hispanic Health and Nutrition Examination Surveys
HIV	Human Immunodeficiency Virus
HIVNET	HIV Network for Prevention Trials
HNPCC	Hereditary Nonpolyposis Colorectal Cancer
IRB	Institutional Review Board
IRS	Intergroup Rhabdomyosarcoma Study
MACS	Multicenter AIDS Cohort Study
MBC	Maryland Brain Center
MGH	Massachusetts General Hospital
MRFIT	Multiple Risk Factor Intervention Trial
MSSM	Mount Sinai School of Medicine
MTS	Mid-America Transplant Services
NBAC	National Bioethics Advisory Commission
NBSB	National Biomonitoring Specimen Bank
NCHS	National Center for Health Statistics
NCI	National Cancer Institute
NEOB	New England Organ Bank
NHANES	National Health and Nutrition Examination Surveys
NHATS	National Human Adipose Tissue Survey
NHES	National Health Examination Surveys
NHL	Non-Hodgkin's lymphoma
NHLBI	National Heart, Lung, and Blood Institute
NHMP	National Human Monitoring Program
NIA	National Institute on Aging
NIAID	National Institute of Allergy and Infectious Disease
NICHD	National Institute of Child Health and Human Development

NIDDK	National Institutes of Diabetes and Digestive and Kidney Diseases
NIGMS	National Institute of General Medical Sciences
NIH	National Institutes of Health
NIMH	National Institute of Mental Health
NINDS	National Institute of Neurological Diseases and Stroke
NIST	National Institute of Standards and Technology
NNRSB	National Neurological Research Specimen Bank
NPF	National Psoriasis Foundation
NPTB	National Psoriasis Tissue Bank
NSABP	National Surgical Adjuvant Breast and Bowel Project
NWTSG	National Wilms Tumor Study Group
NYBC	New York Blood Center
OCT	Optimum cutting temperature
OSU	Ohio State University
PCBs	Polychlorinated biphenyls
PCI	Pittsburgh Cancer Center
PCNA	Proliferating cell nuclear antigen
PCO	Pathology Coordinating Office
PCOS	Polycystic ovary syndrome
POG	Pediatrics Oncology Group
PPH	Primary pulmonary hypertension
PPT	Polyp prevention trial
PSA	Prostate-specific antigen
R&D	Research and development
RMMSC	Rocky Mountain Multiple Sclerosis Center
RTOG	Radiation Therapy Oncology Group
SCOR	Specialized Centers of Research
SEER	Surveillance, Epidemiology, and End Results Program
SHSF	Split hand/split foot

SPORE	Specialized Program of Research Excellence
SWOG	Southwest Oncology Group
TPSR	Tissue Procurement Shared Resource
TRP	Translational Research Program
UAREP	Universities Associated for Research and Education in Pathology
UCCC	University of Colorado Cancer Center
UCSF	The University of California at San Francisco
UMCC	University of Michigan Cancer Center
UNOS	United Network for Organ Sharing
UPMC	University of Pittsburgh Medical Center
VA	Department of Veterans Affairs
VAMC	Veterans Affairs Medical Center
WHI	Women's Health Initiative
WIHS	Women's Interagency HIV Study
WITS	Women and Infants Transmission Study

Chapter One

INTRODUCTION

Human tissues have been stored for a long time. Some institutions in the United States have archived specimens of human tissues that are more than 100 years old. Historically, these stored tissue samples have been used by the biomedical community for educational and research purposes. More recently, stored tissues have played a major role in the understanding and treatment of such diseases as cancer, HIV/AIDS, and heart disease. However, the use and storage of human tissues raise several legal, ethical, and societal issues. Furthermore, as recent and rapid advances in biological and medical research made it possible to analyze DNA from almost any minuscule sample of human tissue, concerns about privacy and informed consent have been raised. Complicating these issues is the paucity of information addressing tissue acquisition, use, and storage.

Once removed, human tissue may serve many beneficial purposes. The most familiar and widespread use of human tissue is in the diagnosis and treatment of illness. Another common use of human tissue is for quality-control purposes in diagnostic and pathologic laboratories. Human tissue is also used for medical and biological research and for medical education and training. Other uses of human tissue include identification, such as in paternity testing, cases of abduction or soldiers missing in action, and forensic purposes in crime cases when biological evidence is available for comparison.

The most common source of tissue is from patients following diagnostic or therapeutic procedures. Tissue specimens may also be taken during autopsies performed to establish the cause of death. In addition, volunteers may donate blood or other tissue for transplantation or research, organs for transplantation, or their bodies for anatomical studies after death. Each specimen of human tissue can be stored in multiple forms, such as slides, paraffin blocks, formalin-fixed, frozen, tissue culture, or extracted DNA.

HISTORICAL PERSPECTIVE

The development of the use of human biological materials for research has been a slow process. Early Egyptians did not study the deceased human body for an explanation of disease and death, though some organs were removed for preservation. The Greeks and Indians cremated their dead without prior examination. The Romans, Chinese, and Muslims all held various taboos and beliefs against opening the body for examination, and thus, no study of human organs or tissues occurred in these societies. Human dissections were also not permitted in Europe during the Middle Ages.

The first real dissections for medical study of disease were carried out around 300 B.C. by Alexandrian physicians Herophilus and Erasistratus. In the late second century A.D., the Greek physician Galen was the first known person to correlate a patient's symptoms with what was found upon an internal examination of the "affected part of the deceased." Greek medicine was essentially the beginning of human medical study based on scientific investigations and observations. Medicine before the Greek advances was almost entirely confined to religious beliefs and rituals. Disease was considered a result of divine interference and human sin, and the maladies of those unlucky individuals were "treated" with spells and prayers.

During the Renaissance, the artists rather than the anatomists were intent on rendering an accurate picture of the human body. Leonardo da Vinci performed dissections and extensive analysis on the human body during the late 1400s and early 1500s. The study of human organs and tissues began to take hold in the nineteenth century. Early biologists viewed their work as a study of the organism. The German pathologist Rudolf Virchow introduced the cellular doctrine, which viewed changes in cells as the basis of the understanding of disease, through his work in pathology and autopsy. In 1838, Theodor Schwann and Matthias Schleiden announced their cell theory that postulated cells as the basic unit of all living tissues.

In 1912, scientists performed an experiment that demonstrated that cells could be kept alive indefinitely if proper conditions were maintained. The advent of transplantation surgery in the mid-twentieth century spurred organ donor programs and organ banks as the technology advanced for specific organs. It was found that without a blood supply, organs would deteriorate rapidly, although cooling could slow the deterioration process somewhat. Blood cells, spermatozoa, and certain other dissociated tissue cells were found to survive subzero freezing indefinitely. Special preserving fluids were shown to prevent cell destruction by ice crystals, but, unfortunately, these fluids have damaging effects if introduced into whole organs. Long-term storage and banking of organs seems unlikely in the near future, because preservation techniques for heart, liver, and lung have not been extensively studied (the kidney can be pre-served up to 72 hours).

Several historical examples have demonstrated the value of archived tissue samples. For example, research in tracking viruses and studies tracing the pathology of a particular disease have been extremely beneficial to medical research (NBAC, 1999). A recent case involved the rediscovery of slides stored by Alois Alzheimer and the confirmation of his original diagnosis by histological and genetic analysis (Graeber et al., 1997; 1998). Slides of the first brain known to have Alzheimer's disease were stored in 1906, and a paper was published in 1907 describing the disease. The search for the brain of patient Auguste D. began when her original hospital file was found in 1996 at an institute at the University of Frankfurt. In 1998, more than 250 slides of Auguste's brain were found in a basement at the University of Munich, where Alois Alzheimer worked at the time of her death. The reexamination of the slides clarified the definitive pathologic diagnosis of Alzheimer's disease.

TYPES OF TISSUE/ORGAN BANKS

Tissue collections vary considerably, ranging from formal repositories to the informal storage of blood or tissue specimens in a researcher's freezer. The form in which the tissue is stored can also vary widely, including solid organs, sections of organs, histology slides, cells, and DNA. Large collections include archived pathology samples, autopsy material, and tissue biopsies from diag-nostic tests. These tissue samples are stored at military facilities, the National Institutes of Health and its sponsored facilities, other federal agencies, state collection agencies (e.g., state forensic DNA banks and newborn screening lab-oratories), diagnostic pathology and cytology laboratories, university- and hospital-based research laboratories, commercial enterprises, and nonprofit organizations.

USES OF TISSUE/ORGAN BANKS FOR BIOMEDICAL RESEARCH

A common use of stored tissues was to correlate changes in structure or appearance of a tissue with a diagnosis of a particular disease. Pathology exams were performed broadly with what could be seen by the naked eye and even-tually with the light microscope. As the understanding of science advanced, tis-sue analysis was reduced to a smaller scale. Molecular biology and genetics research has minimized the need for viably stored tissue. Frozen tissue, paraf-fin blocks, or formalin-fixed tissue is sufficient for the study of protein and gene expression and genetic mutations. Research of tissue samples has evolved toward a much smaller scale, where once a large portion of an organ may have been required for study, a single slice or a million cells is now more than sufficient to answer a researcher's question. Thus, a single freezer could store a life-time of research samples on a particular tissue or disease.

Different areas of research that routinely use tissue samples include studies of gene or protein expression, initial analysis of tissues affected by a newly discovered viral or bacterial pathogen, studies of changes in genetic sequences over time or in different populations, genetic linkage studies in normal and affected populations to narrow the location of the mutant gene, and analysis of cell structure in affected and normal tissue. The older a tissue bank is, the more valuable it may be to ascertain changes over time as environmental or societal shifts occur. The need to achieve statistical significance requires large sample numbers, and thus researchers may need to use tissue samples from a number of different banks. The ongoing need for tissue samples in research calls for a handbook, such as this, to facilitate the process of finding particular tissues for research. Both public and private entities use tissue samples for both academic and commercial enterprises. The savings in time and money of avoiding collection of tissues for each new research study is invaluable to the researcher in an environment where both are scarce.

AN INVENTORY OF TISSUE SOURCES IN THE UNITED STATES

To date, no central database captures information about stored tissue samples. To obtain a better understanding of the magnitude of existing archives, the National Bioethics Advisory Commission (NBAC) initially requested information from RAND about stored tissue samples in the United States. The purpose of the report was to collect for the first time in a single document information about tissue storage in the United States. Although it was not meant to be a comprehensive inventory, the report identified the major sources of stored tissue. This handbook is an extension of the NBAC commissioned report and is meant to serve as an inventory resource of stored tissue samples in the United States. The abundance of such samples in the United States is essentially useless to scientific investigators unless they are aware of its existence and its availability. The report as well as this handbook attempts to provide information about several aspects of stored tissue samples by addressing the following questions:

1. Where are tissues stored? (e.g., repositories, pathology laboratories, blood banks)

2. How many tissue samples are stored at each institution?

3. Who are the sources of stored tissue samples? (e.g., patients, volunteers)

4. Why were the tissue samples originally collected? (e.g., diagnostic purposes, research)

5. For what purposes have the stored tissues been used? (e.g., cancer research, gene mapping)

6. Who has access to the samples? (e.g., researchers, insurers, employers)

7. How are the tissue samples stored (e.g., paraffin blocks, slides, frozen tissue) and for how long? (e.g., months, years, indefinitely)

8. What identifying information is kept with the tissues? (e.g., patient's name or medical record number).

We intend this handbook to serve the research community as a comprehensive reference source of tissue banks in the United States and to facilitate the distribution of tissues for individual research projects.

DEFINITIONS

Several terms are used in this handbook that need further definition:

> *Human tissue* is defined as including everything from subcellular structures like DNA, to cells, tissue (bone, muscle, connective tissue, and skin), organs (e.g., liver, bladder, heart, kidney), blood, gametes (sperm and ova), embryos, fetal tissue, and waste (urine, feces, sweat, hair and nail clippings, shed epithelial cells, placenta).

> This handbook attempts to count both the number of *cases* from which stored tissues are derived as well as the number of *specimens* generated from each case. For example, when a patient enters the hospital for a biopsy, the resulting tissue is accessioned in the pathology department as a single case. However, that single biopsy may generate several specimens, including a number of slides, paraffin blocks, and frozen specimens. When portions of specimens are distributed to researchers, the researcher is receiving a *sample* of that specimen. For example, a specimen of frozen brain tissue from a case of Alzheimer's disease may provide a number of researchers with samples for use in genetic linkage studies.

> The term *DNA bank* refers to a facility that stores extracted DNA, transformed cell lines, frozen blood or tissue, or biological samples for future DNA analysis. Specimens are usually stored with some form of individual identification for later retrieval. *DNA databanks* are repositories of genetic information obtained from the analysis of DNA samples, sometimes referred to as *DNA profiles*. The genetic information is usually stored in computerized form with individual identifiers.

> *Graduate medical education (GME) programs* are the primary means of medical education beyond the four-year medical school training received by all physicians. GME programs are usually referred to as residency

programs and are based in hospitals or other health-care institutions, some of which do and some of which do not have formal relationships with medical schools. *GME teaching institutions* include medical schools; U.S. armed forces hospitals; Veterans Affairs medical centers; the Public Health Service; state, county, and city hospitals; nonprofit institutions; and health maintenance organizations.

DATA COLLECTION

For this handbook, collections of stored tissue samples were identified through several sources: a literature review of papers about tissue banks and DNA banks; searches of the worldwide web; searches of RAND's RaDiUS database and NIH's CRISP database to identify federally funded sources of stored tissue; and personal communications and consultation with experts. Several papers served as valuable sources of information on DNA banks and DNA databanks, including forensic DNA banks and the Department of Defense DNA Specimen Repository for Remains Identification. Information contained in numerous Internet Web sites for several tissue banks, organ banks, umbilical cord blood banks, sperm and embryo banks, and longitudinal studies was also used. Relevant Web sites appear in Appendix I and Appendix J of this report. RAND's RaDiUS database provided information about government, university, non-profit, and commercially based tissue repositories. Finally, a substantial amount of information was obtained through personal communications with knowledgeable sources in the field, including pathologists, relevant people at several tissue banks, and experts who have published papers on the subject of stored tissue samples.

RaDiUS

RAND's Research and Development in the United States (RaDiUS) database is a comprehensive, real-time accounting of federal research and development (R&D) activities and spending. RaDiUS allows users to see the total R&D investment by all federal agencies, to compare the level of R&D investment in specific areas of science and technology across all federal agencies, or to examine the details of research investments within a specific agency. RaDiUS was searched using proximity and wildcard searches for combinations of different search terms, including "tissue(s)," "bank(s)," "repository(ies)," "blood," "DNA," and "cell(s)."

ESTIMATE OF CASES ACCESSIONED AT GRADUATE MEDICAL EDUCATION TEACHING INSTITUTIONS

Two techniques were used to estimate the total number of cases accessioned per year at all GME institutions and the number of tissues stored at each institution. The first estimate used information found in the American Medical Association's Graduate Medical Education Directory 1997–1998 about residency programs in pathology at GME institutions (American Medical Association, 1997). However, not all pathology specialties yielded information. Therefore, a second estimate was made from information obtained from several chairs of pathology departments attending the Universities Associated for Research and Education in Pathology (UAREP) conference hosted by the Federation of American Societies for Experimental Biology (FASEB).

An analysis was performed (see Figure 2.1) to estimate the total number of cases accessioned per year at all GME teaching institutions in the pathology spe-

i = state (e.g., New York, Massachusetts, Virginia)
j = specialty (e.g., anatomic, forensic, pediatric)
k = procedure (e.g., autopsy, surgical pathology, cytology)
α = duration of the program in years

X_{ij} = number of programs by state i and specialty j

Y_{ij} = number of residents by state i and specialty j

$Z_j = \sum_i X_{ij}$ = total number of programs by specialty

$W_j = \sum_i Y_{ij}$ = total number of residents by specialty

$S_{jk} = \dfrac{\text{number of tissue samples examined by specialty } j,\ \text{procedure } k \text{ per resident}}{\text{duration of program in years } \alpha}$ = number of tissue samples examined by specialty j, procedure k per year per resident

$T_{jk} = W_j * S_{jk}$ = total number of samples required for all residents to see by specialty j and procedure k per year

$U_j = \sum_k T_{jk}$ = total number of samples required for all residents to see by specialty j per year

$V = \sum_j U_j$ = total number samples per year

Figure 2.1- **Mathematical Model for Cases Accessioned at GME Teaching Institutions**

cialties of anatomic and clinical pathology, dermatopathology, forensic pathology, neuropathology, and pediatric pathology. This calculation was based on the number of GME pathology programs in each specialty (Z_j); the number of resident positions open in these programs for the academic year (W_j); the recommended number of cases per program to meet the training requirements of the residents (T_{jk}); and the duration of the program in years (α). A mathematical model showing the calculations used is shown below. An estimate of the number of cases and specimens accessioned in cytopathology and hematopathology programs was obtained by averaging the number of cases and specimens reported on various GME teaching institutions' Internet Web sites.

Chairs of pathology departments attending the UAREP meeting were asked several questions about the pathology departments at their institutions. Information from 10 pathology chairs was obtained about the size of their institution, the number of cases accessioned per year, the age of the oldest tissues archived, how long the tissue samples are stored, what identifying information is kept with the tissues, and who has access to the samples. This information was used to calculate ranges and averages of hospital size and number of cases accessioned.

ORGANIZATION OF HANDBOOK

This book is organized into sections based on the type of institution where the tissue is stored. Chapter Three describes large tissue banks, repositories, and core facilities, including those that are federally funded, those at research universities and academic medical centers, and commercial and nonprofit entities. Chapter Four describes tumor registries and the types of data and information they collect. Chapter Five describes longitudinal studies and research projects that simultaneously create tissue collections. Chapter Six describes human tissue specimens collected through hospital pathology departments—the oldest and largest source of human tissues in the United States. The remaining three chapters describe state screening laboratories and forensic DNA banks, cryopreservation facilities and storage banks, and private and public umbilical cord blood banks, respectively. Detailed appendixes list addresses (D, F, H, and I) and Web sites (J) of all tissue banks described in the handbook, as well as many more too numerous to describe individually. We intend this handbook to serve the research community as a comprehensive reference source of tissue banks in the United States and to facilitate the distribution of tissues for individual research projects.

Chapter Three

LARGE TISSUE BANKS, REPOSITORIES, AND CORE FACILITIES

Large tissue banks and repositories exist in almost every sector of the scientific and medical communities, including the military, the federal government, universities and academic medical centers, commercial enterprises, and nonprofit organizations. In addition, several universities have established core tissue banking facilities to support both their own research and collaborations with other universities. These large tissue banks, repositories, and core facilities are major sources of human tissue for biomedical research.

MILITARY FACILITIES

The military maintains two of the largest tissue repositories in the world. The National Pathology Repository and the Department of Defense (DoD) DNA Specimen Repository for Remains Identification are housed within the Armed Forces Institute of Pathology (AFIP). The AFIP is responsible for maintaining a central laboratory of pathology for consultation and diagnosis of pathologic tissue for DoD, other federal agencies, and civilian pathologists. The AFIP also conducts research in pathology, trains enlisted personnel in histopathology and related techniques, and offers more than 50 pathology education courses for medical, dental, and veterinary personnel.

National Pathology Repository

The National Pathology Repository, located at the AFIP, is the largest and most comprehensive collection of pathology material in the world. Since 1917, the Pathology Repository has collected more than 2.5 million cases comprising more than 50 million microscopic slides, 30 million paraffin tissue blocks, 12 million preserved wet tissue specimens, and associated written records. The Pathology Repository accessions approximately 50,000 cases annually, with 53,384 cases accessioned in fiscal year (FY) 1996, and 51,908 in 1997. In addition, approximately 40,000 cytology cases are sent for primary diagnosis annually but are not accessioned (only cytology cases sent for second opinions are accessioned). During 1993, approximately 10,000 of the cases were cancers and 8,000 were benign neoplasms, with the balance representing the entire spectrum of human disease. Material is stored permanently unless a specific request comes from the contributor or other authorized individual to return or release the material.

The AFIP accepts cases from all Army, Navy, and Air Force medical facilities and investigative agencies. The AFIP also serves as the central laboratory of pathology for the DoD and certain other federal agencies, such as the Public Health Service and the Justice Department. In addition, the AFIP serves as a Veterans Affairs Special Reference Laboratory for Pathology and maintains a special registry of former prisoners of war. Civilian and foreign contributions are accepted from pathologists (or clinicians functioning as pathologists) through the Civilian Consultation program. Cases represent both sexes, all races/ethnicities, and all ages and come from contributors worldwide.

Cases are sent to the AFIP for a variety of reasons. The majority of cases are submitted to the AFIP because the contributor wants a second opinion regarding the diagnosis. Some are forwarded as part of established peer-review and quality-assurance programs. DoD regulations require some military cases to be forwarded, such as forensic cases and cases subject to litigation. Other cases are submitted because they are rare and could be used by the AFIP in their research and education missions. In addition, cases have been submitted over the years for specific purposes, such as to study particular diseases or to answer current and future research questions (for example, sera from Gulf War veterans).

All submitted case material is coded by pathological diagnosis and is identified by an AFIP accession number. The source name, Social Security number, date of birth, age, sex, and race are stored if provided by the contributing pathologist. Any medical history provided is stored in the case folder and on an optical disk imaging system. The source address is not routinely provided or stored but is obtained on occasion for follow-up studies. Likewise, the original consent remains a matter between the patient and the clinician and is not routinely provided to AFIP by the contributing pathologist. The submitting pathologist's name and address and the source's surgical identification numbers are also stored.

All research protocols using Pathology Repository stored material or data are reviewed by the AFIP's Institutional Review Board (IRB). Research involving patient follow-up, and thus requiring identifying information, is reviewed at a full meeting of the IRB prior to approval. Other than for research involving follow-up, original sources of material are not notified. If an unexpected disease or abnormality is discovered, the contributing pathologist is notified, then it is up to the pathologist to contact the patient. Otherwise, current AFIP policy requires that material be made anonymous before release to outside investigators.

The main functions of the Pathology Repository are consultation, education, and research in pathology. The Pathology Repository also loans pathologic material to assist in patient treatment, for research, or for litigation. Requests for loan of material or provision of data for research purposes require submission and approval of a research protocol. Requests from individuals or organizations other than the original contributor must be accompanied by a properly executed authorization signed by the patient or designated representative. Pathologic specimens stored at the Pathology Repository can be used to study unusual tumors or as part of a public health surveillance system to study emerging infectious diseases or trends in disease progression. For example, samples in the repository have been used to identify and date tissues harboring genomic material of the Human Immunodeficiency Virus (HIV) obtained before the availability of HIV testing and before the worldwide spread of the HIV infection.

DoD DNA Specimen Repository for Remains Identification

The DoD DNA Specimen Repository for Remains Identification is the world's largest DNA bank. As of September 1999, the DNA Repository has received more than 2.8 million DNA specimens. Specimens come into the DNA Repository at a rate of 10,000 per day, and the tally (database) is updated every seven seconds. It is estimated that by 2001 the DNA Repository will contain approximately 3.5 million samples. All DNA specimens will be maintained for 50 years before being destroyed. However, donors may request that their specimens be destroyed following the conclusion of their military service obligation or other applicable relationship to DoD.

Since June 1992, DoD has required all military inductees, and all active-duty and reserve personnel to provide blood and saliva samples for its DNA Specimen Repository at the time of enlistment, reenlistment, annual physical, or preparation for operational deployment (McEwen, 1997). The DNA Repository also contains samples from civilians and foreign nationals who work with the U.S. military in arenas of conflict. Three DNA specimens are collected from each person: a bloodstain card (stored in a pouch in the service member's medical record), a second bloodstain card, and a buccal swab (stored at the DNA Specimen Repository). The blood is placed on special cards with the service member's Social Security number, date of birth, and branch of service designated on the front side of the card and a fingerprint, a bar code, and signature attesting to the validity of the sample on the reverse. The bloodstain card stored at the DNA Repository is placed in a vacuum-sealed bag and frozen at −20°C. The buccal swab is fixed in isopropanol and stored at room temperature. DNA will be extracted from the specimens in the repository only when it is needed for remains identification.

The DNA Repository, along with the Armed Forces DNA Identification Laboratory (AFDIL), make up the DoD DNA Registry. The purpose of the DNA Registry is to identify the remains of soldiers killed in combat or missing in action. High-velocity weapons often destroy any chances of using fingerprints or dental records, but DNA can almost always be used to identify remains. Most times the armed forces can identify the dead based on rosters, but DNA identification provides closure for the family and biological proof of death required by life insurance companies. The military's policy ensures that specimens can be used only for remains identification and routine quality control, except for cases subpoenaed for the investigation or prosecution of a felony. The specimens cannot be used without consent for any other purpose, such as paternity suits or genetic testing. In addition, the specimens are considered confidential medical information, and military regulations and federal law exist to cover any privacy concerns.

NATIONAL INSTITUTES OF HEALTH

The National Institutes of Health (NIH), founded in 1930, consists of 24 separate Institutes, Centers, and Divisions. NIH is the principal health research agency of the federal government. It is one of the eight health agencies of the Public Health Service, which is part of the U.S. Department of Health and Human Services. The mission of NIH is to protect and improve human health. To accomplish its mission, NIH conducts and supports basic, applied, and clinical health services research aimed at understanding the processes underlying human health and acquiring new knowledge to help prevent, diagnose, and treat human diseases and disabilities. In 1999, the NIH budget was more than $15.65 billion. The extramural program, which accounts for approximately 80–85 percent of NIH's total budget, awards grants to researchers at universities, medical schools, hospitals, small businesses, and research institutions across the country, while the intramural program, which represents approximately 11 percent of the budget, supports research and training of scientists at NIH. NIH is probably the single highest funder of extramural tissue and data resources for basic, applied, and clinical research. Some of the institutes at NIH that support tissue banks include the National Cancer Institute, the National Institute of Allergy and Infectious Disease, the National Heart, Lung, and Blood Institute, the National Institute of Mental Health, the National Institute on Aging, the

National Institute of Environmental Health Sciences, and the National Institute of Diabetes and Digestive and Kidney Diseases.

National Cancer Institute

The National Cancer Institute (NCI), the largest of NIH's biomedical research institutes and centers, has coordinated the U.S. government's cancer research program since 1937. Through both its extramural and intramural programs, the NCI supports research on all aspects of cancer prevention, detection, diagnosis, and treatment. In addition, the NCI supports several tissue and data resources for cancer research, including the NCI Cooperative Human Tissue Network, the NCI Clinical Trials Cooperative Group Human Tissue Resources, the NCI Cooperative Breast Cancer Tissue Resource, the NCI Breast Cancer Specimen and Data Information System, the NCI Cooperative Family Registry for Breast Cancer Studies and NCI Cooperative Family Registry for Colorectal Cancer Studies, and the NCI AIDS Malignancy Bank.

The NCI supports a great number of other tissue banks and collection systems. Among the many NCI-funded tissue collections are breast and prostate cancer and HIV/AIDS. These tissue collections may vary in their specific objectives and goals, but, overall, the tissues are collected for the advancement of knowledge and development of clinical applications in a particular field.

NCI Cooperative Human Tissue Network. The Cooperative Human Tissue Network (CHTN), supported by the NCI since 1987, provides biomedical researchers access to fresh surgical or biopsy specimens of normal, benign, precancerous, and cancerous human tissues. The CHTN is a tissue collection system and not a tissue bank. Only very rare specimens that are difficult to obtain are stored to anticipate future requests. Except for a collection of frozen tissue from rare pediatric tumors, banked specimens are generally not stored for more than one year. Normally, the specimens are obtained prospectively to fill specific researcher requests. Five member institutions coordinate the collection and distribution of tissues across the United States and Canada.[1] Tissues are provided by the CHTN only for research purposes and cannot be sold or used for commercial purposes. The intent of the CHTN is to encourage research using human tissue for the good of the public rather than for private gain.

During the first nine years of its operation, the CHTN supplied more than 100,000 specimens to approximately 600 investigators. CHTN tissues have been used widely in cancer research for both basic and developmental studies,

---

[1]The five regional divisions are the Eastern Division, the Midwestern Division, the Southern Division, the Western Division, and the Pediatric Division, which provides samples of childhood tumors nationwide through the Children's Cancer Study Group.

including molecular biology, immunology, and genetics. Researchers have used these tissues to study mutations of protooncogenes in human tumors and the role of growth factors in cancer and to isolate new cancer genes. More than 2,000 publications have resulted from studies using CHTN tissues.

The CHTN obtains tissues from routine surgical resections and autopsies. Tissues from both adult and pediatric patients represent all organ systems, as well as blood and other body fluids. Specimens are collected according to the individual investigator's protocol and may be preserved as fresh, fixed or frozen, slides, or paraffin blocks. The CHTN was designed for basic research studies not requiring clinical follow-up information. Each specimen is given a unique identifier, and a link is maintained by the parent institution for quality-control purposes. Only minimal demographic data is provided with each specimen. Other information routinely provided with the specimen includes pathology reports and histological characterization.

Participating CHTN institutions include the University of Alabama at Birmingham, University of Pennsylvania Medical Center, the Ohio State University Medical Center, Case Western Reserve University, and Children's Hospital of Columbus.

NCI Clinical Trials Cooperative Group Human Tissue Resources. The NCI Clinical Trials Cooperative Group (CTCG) is a program of national networks that conduct large-scale, multi-institutional clinical trials supported by the Cancer Therapy Evaluation Program, Division of Cancer Treatment and Diagnosis. The primary goal of CTCG is the definitive evaluation of clinical treatment programs. Currently, the groups conduct approximately 400 clinical trials, evaluating approximately 20,000 patients a year. The large amount of patient data collected annually through these trials and the large-scale collection of biologic specimens with clinical and outcome data provide researchers with a rich resource of specimens for correlative studies. The network member groups that maintain tissue banks are briefly described below.

Pediatric Oncology Group. The Pediatric Oncology Group (POG), established in 1980, is a consortium of 39 full member institutions, 48 affiliate, 12 consortia, and 9 CCOP institutions. This consortium has pooled its patient resources and scientific expertise to study the natural history of childhood cancer, develop and compare effective therapeutic regimens, and investigate the toxicity and efficacy of new anticancer agents in the treatment of childhood cancer. Many of the members are funded through the NCI. Since 1980, nearly 50,000 children have been enrolled in pediatric cancer research studies. Several tissue banks have been established to provide qualified investigators with tissue and cells for studies focused on childhood cancers. For example, the Acute Lymphoblastic Leukemia (ALL) Cell Bank (Stanford University, California) has collected thousands of frozen cell suspensions from bone marrow extractions from ALL patients. The cell bank collects and stores approximately 600 new samples each year. Other POG-maintained tissue banks are listed below:

Pediatric Oncology Group—Hodgkin's Disease Cell Bank *(Wake Forest University, North Carolina)*

Pediatric Oncology Group—Germ Cell Tumor Bank *(University of Alabama, Birmingham, Alabama)*

Pediatric Oncology Group—Lymphoid Relapse Cell Bank *(MCSD Medical Center, California)*

Pediatric Oncology Group—Neuroblastoma Tumor Bank *(Children's Memorial Hospital, Illinois)*

Pediatric Oncology Group—NHL Cell Bank *(University of Massachusetts Medical School, Massachusetts)*

Pediatric Oncology Group—Hepatoblastoma Biology Study and Tissue Bank *(University of Texas Southwestern Medical Center, Texas)*

Pediatric Oncology Group—AML Cell Bank *(St. Jude Children's Research Hospital, Tennessee)*

Pediatric Oncology Group—CNS Tumor Bank *(Duke University, North Carolina)*

Pediatric Oncology Group—Sarcoma Cell Bank (*Dana-Farber Cancer Institute, Massachusetts*)

Gynecologic Oncology Group Tissue Bank. The Gynecologic Oncology Group (GOG) Tissue Bank, supported by the NCI, provides malignant, benign, and normal ovarian and cervical tissue from almost 3,200 patients for molecular biology studies of gynecologic tumors. The specimens are stored as snap-frozen specimens, formalin-fixed sections, OCT embedded primary tumors, touch imprint slides, and patient serum collected prior to surgery. Currently, specimens are stored dating back five years. Each case is given a unique identifier, and a link is kept at the GOG Tissue Bank. The link provides a one-way flow of information for research purposes. Clinical information is provided with each case and may include patient age and race in addition to the institutional pathology and operative reports.

Specimens obtained from patients in clinical trials at approximately 76 participating institutions are stored centrally at the Children's Hospital Research Foundation in Columbus, Ohio. The GOG Tissue Bank is ideal for clinical correlative studies to identify those factors that place patients with ovarian carcinoma at high risk for treatment failure independent of such traditional variables as stage, grade and cell type. A total of 52 projects, focusing mainly on the molecular genetics underlying gynecologic malignancies, have utilized this resource.

Intergroup Rhabdomyosarcoma Tissue Bank. The Intergroup Rhabdomyosarcoma Study (IRS) was initiated in 1972 and is a collaborative multidisciplinary study carried out by the Children's Cancer Group (CCG) and the POG. The IRS was designed to answer therapeutic, clinical, and laboratory questions about rhabdomyosarcoma. Eligible patients in CCG and POG institutions are enrolled in IRS protocols. Four major study protocols have taken place, and between 600 and 1,000 patients have been enrolled in each protocol. Tissue samples from patients in many of these protocols have been collected and stored in the Intergroup Rhabdomyosarcoma Tissue Bank for future study.

Cancer and Leukemia Group B. The Cancer and Leukemia Group B (CALGB) was founded in 1955 and is a national clinical research group sponsored by the NCI. CALGB consists of 31 university medical centers, more than 185 community hospitals, and more than 3,000 physicians. CALGB seeks to conduct clinical research studies aimed at reducing the morbidity and mortality from cancer, to relate the biological characteristics of cancer to clinical outcomes, and to develop new strategies for the early detection and prevention of cancer. CALGB research focuses on six diseases: leukemia, lymphoma, breast cancer, lung cancer, gastrointestinal malignancies, and prostate cancer.

The CALGB maintains a leukemia tissue bank at the Arthur G. James Cancer Hospital and Research Institute in Columbus, Ohio. Tissue specimens from study participants are collected from newly diagnosed patients with acute or chronic leukemia or myelodysplastic syndrome who are entered into a CALGB protocol for previously untreated patients. The specimens are archived for future investigations. Bone marrow, blood, and buccal swabs are collected from patients. Requests for tissue will be reviewed for scientific merit, strength of the analytical techniques, and track record of the investigator, among other criteria.

Children's Cancer Group. The Children's Cancer Group (CCG) was founded in 1955 and is a national cooperative research organization devoted to the development of new treatments and cures for childhood cancers. CCG conducts research on the biology of these cancers, their etiology, and long-term followup of cured patients into adult life. In 1990, the National Childhood Cancer Foundation was established as the fiscal agent of CCG. More than 2,500 pediatric cancer specialists are CCG members at more than 115 pediatric medical centers in the United States, Canada, and Australia. CCG's main priority is to facilitate the transition of new biological findings into clinical trials for treatments of childhood cancer.

Tissue specimens are collected from study participants and stored for future investigations. The CCG maintains a solid tumor tissue bank, an AML tissue bank, and an ALL tissue bank.

National Wilms Tumor Study Group. The National Wilms Tumor Study Group (NWTSG) was established in 1969, and POG and CCG member institutions participate as part of their study groups. The NWTSG seeks to increase the survival rate of children with Wilms tumor and other renal tumors, to study the long-term outcome of children who have been treated successfully for Wilms tumor, to identify adverse effects of treatment for Wilms tumor, to conduct epidemiological and biological studies of Wilms tumor, and to disseminate information regarding successful treatment strategies of Wilms tumor.

More than 100 pediatric oncology treatment centers are involved in NWTSG therapeutic studies. Approximately 440 patients are enrolled annually into NWTSG studies. A tissue bank is maintained for tissue specimens collected from NWTSG study participants for future research.

Radiation Therapy Oncology Group. The Radiation Therapy Oncology Group (RTOG), established in 1968, has received funding from the NCI since 1971. RTOG is a national cooperative cancer study group that conducts multicenter clinical trials that integrate surgical, radiotherapeutic, and chemotherapeutic treatments. Since its inception, the RTOG has activated 271 protocols and accrued almost 56,000 patients in its cooperative group studies. Close to 300 radiation oncology departments in North America are members of the RTOG, which has its headquarters at the American College of Radiology in Philadelphia, Pennsylvania. In 1996, RTOG created the Translational Research Program (TRP), which coordinates RTOG's basic science committees, including the Tumor Repository.

In 1993, a frozen tumor tissue repository was established at Fox Chase Cancer Center to provide access to frozen tissue for use in correlative and translational studies. The frozen tumor repository collects 3–5 frozen tissue fragments per case from phase III protocols of cervical, lung, head and neck, esophageal, and anal cancers. Currently, the frozen tumor repository contains more than 290 specimens from approximately 70 different tumors (cases). About two-thirds of the specimens are from cervical cancer, and the next most abundant specimens are from head and neck tumors.

Because of technological advances allowing the analysis of tumor markers in paraffinized tissue removed from tumors, the RTOG began archiving paraffin blocks and tissues from all RTOG phase III trials in 1995. Phase III protocols for cancer of the prostate, bladder, lung, head and neck, esophagus, and malignant glioma were modified to contain a request for blocks or unstained slides on each patient. The patient consent form was modified to allow tissues to be stored and used for future research. These tissues are used for population-based studies but not for patient-related issues. Investigators performing research on RTOG specimens lack access to clinical information that might allow patient identification or linkage to treatment and demographics. A central processing site for all blocks and unstained slides was established in February 1996 and funded by the NCI in November 1996. The fixed tissue repository was moved to Latter-Day Saints Hospital in March 1997. Currently, the RTOG has approximately 4,400 cases stored at a central repository in Salt Lake City, Utah, and is accruing about 1,500 cases per year.

Eastern Cooperative Oncology Group. The Eastern Cooperative Oncology Group (ECOG), established in 1955, is supported by the NCI. ECOG is an international organization with more than 365 university and community-based hospitals and practices and more than 5,000 participating scientists and health-care professionals, including physicians, statisticians, nurses, clinical research associates, and pharmacists. ECOG's primary functions include conducting clinical trials that compare new therapeutic approaches to standard therapies, assessing dose and toxicity levels, and determining response rates of experimental therapies. In addition to clinical trials, ECOG conducts studies in cancer control and prevention and performs translational research. ECOG's overall goal is to improve the care of patients with cancer.

Tissue banking is an integral part of the laboratory science effort of ECOG. ECOG maintains four tissue banking facilities, a solid tumor tissue bank, a myeloma tissue bank, a leukemia cell bank, and an immunologic tumor repository. In January 1997, ECOG moved the solid tumor tissue bank and disbursement facility from the ECOG Operations Office in Boston, Massachusetts, to the Pathology Coordinating Office (PCO) in Evanston, Illinois. The new facility consists of 750 square feet of space—a 500-square-foot laboratory, a specially designed 250-square-foot walk-in cold room for storage of paraffin-embedded tissue blocks and slides, and a –80°C freezer for storage of bone marrow and DNA. The ECOG-PCO is responsible for acquisition, storage, data entry, tissue processing, and quality assurance of solid tumors and lymphomas. The ECOG-PCO stores both retrospective, archived fixed tissues (blocks and slides) and prospectively collected tissues (blocks, slides, frozen tissues, etc.). Tissue samples will never be discarded from the bank, and great efforts will be made to maintain at least a portion of all samples indefinitely. Tissues will be returned to their home institutions for storage if the ECOG-PCO bank ever closes. In 1995, the solid tumor bank contained 3,000 paraffin-embedded blocks and 15,000 slides with an estimated accrual rate of 3,000 blocks per year. The ECOG-PCO bank also stores specimens for three other Cancer Cooperative Groups—the Southwest Oncology Group (SWOG), the Cancer and Leukemia Group B (CALGB), and the Radiation Therapy Oncology Group (RTOG).

Southwest Oncology Group. The Southwest Oncology Group (SWOG) was first organized as a pediatric oncology group in 1956 but has evolved into an adult multidisease, multimodality, clinical research organization. SWOG is primarily funded by the NCI and includes 34 full member institutions; 26 Community Clinical Oncology Programs (CCOP) institutions, including seven minority-based CCOPs; 23 urologic cancer outreach programs; 25 high-priority program members; and a network of approximately 1,000 Cooperative Group Outreach Programs (CGOPs) investigators at 291 affiliate hospitals. Approximately 3,500 oncologists are members of SWOG and actively participate in the enrollment of patients to oncology protocols. Participants in SWOG study protocols are in excess of 8,000 per year. Tissue samples collected from participants are stored in the SWOG National Tissue Repository for future use by approved investigators in the field of oncology. For example, the Intergroup Breast Tissue Bank has more than 4,000 breast tissue specimens and estimates that more than 8,000 additional specimens from nine study protocols will be collected.

National Surgical Adjuvant Breast and Bowel Project. The National Surgical Adjuvant Breast and Bowel Project (NSABP) was established in 1971 and is primarily supported by the NCI. The NSABP is a cooperative group that conducts clinical trials in breast and colorectal cancer research. Currently, almost 300 participating medical centers in the United States and more than 6,000 physicians, nurses, and other medical professionals conduct NSABP research. In 1997, NSABP treatment trial members enrolled more than 3,000 breast and colorectal patients in seven treatment trials. The NSABP has collected malignant breast tissue samples from 10,000 patients enrolled in NSABP trials. These specimens are available for confirmatory studies for potential therapeutic response variables and limited nongenetic studies.

NCI Breast Cancer Specimen and Data Information System. The NCI has developed a national information database of breast cancer resources to help investigators studying breast cancer identify sources of biological specimens for use in their research. The NCI Breast Cancer Specimen and Data Information System contains information about 14 breast tissue banks. This database does not represent an exhaustive national listing of all facilities holding breast cancer tissue. However, by centralizing information on biological specimens, this database promotes access to breast tissue specimens and facilitates collaboration among basic, clinical and epidemiologic researchers. Table 3.1 summarizes the information contained in the NCI Breast Cancer Specimen and Data Information System.

Cumulatively, the 14 breast tissue banks in the NCI database contain more than 130,000 cases of breast cancer–related specimens and data, with banks ranging in size from 48 cases to approximately 101,000 cases (see Table 3.1). Three of

Table 3.1

NCI Breast Cancer Specimen and Data Information System

Resource	Number of Specimens/Tissue Type(s)	Other Data	Limitations	Consent
Baylor SPORE—Familial Breast Cancer Registry and Gene Bank Alkek N550, MS 600 One Baylor Plaza Houston, TX 77030 Ph. 713-798-1600 Fax: 713-198-1642	6 frozen and 42 paraffin-embedded malignant breast cancer specimens Blood or blood products Frozen and paraffin-embedded malignant tissue	Demographic Clinical Outcome	Proposals reviewed and approved by Baylor SPORE Executive Committee, and collaboration is required	Specific patient consent form for research use of breast cancer-related specimens
Baylor SPORE—National Breast Cancer Tissue Resource Alkek N550, MS 600 One Baylor Plaza Houston, TX 77030 Ph. 713-798-1600 Fax: 713-198-1642	151,320 biopsy specimens from about 101,000 cases of breast cancer Frozen malignant tissue	Demographic Clinical Outcome	Proposals reviewed and approved by Baylor SPORE Executive Committee, and collaboration is required	Standard hospital consent
Dana Farber Cancer Institute 44 Binney St. Boston, MA 02115 Ph. 617-632-5189 Fax: 617-632-5189	225 invasive breast cancer cases aged 32 and under Cell lines Genomic DNA Plasma Viable frozen cells	Demographic Clinical Other	Outside advisory committee prioritizes requests for specimens and risk factor data; no identifying information provided. Tissue samples are available for detection of p53, BRCA1, and additional inherited breast cancer susceptibility genes and studies of gene-environmental interactions Costs associated with generating and delivering all specimens requested	Not applicable since data provided is unidentified

Table 3.1- continued

Resource	Number of Specimens/ Tissue Type(s)	Other Data	Limitations	Consent
Duke University Box 3873 Duke University Medical Center Durham, NC 27710	>1,400 blood and tissue samples in inventory (50 fresh and 100 frozen tissues per year) Blood or blood products Fresh and frozen malignant, benign, and normal tissue	Demographic Clinical Outcome	Use by Duke researchers is high and has priority, otherwise collaboration is required	Standard hospital consent
Georgetown University Medical Center and Lombardi Cancer Center and SPORE 3900 Reservoir Rd., N.W. Washington, D.C. 20007 Ph. 202-687-2904 Fax: 202-687-8935	~200 cases per year of paraffin-embedded tissue since the mid-1970s (each case has from 3–30 tissue blocks) Blood or blood products Frozen and paraffin-embedded malignant, benign, and normal tissue	Demographic Clinical Outcome	Use of some samples restricted for use by Lombardi Cancer Center investigators, otherwise collaboration is required	Standard hospital consent
National Cancer Institute of Canada—Manitoba Breast Tumor Bank 100 Olivia St. Winnipeg Manitoba R3E OV9 Canada Ph. 204-787-1446 Fax: 204-783-6875	Malignant: >2,000 frozen and >2,000 paraffin-embedded Normal: 100 frozen and 100 paraffin-embedded	Demographic Clinical Other	Acknowledgment of bank in publication required Use of material restricted to studies proposed Data limited to information requested at outset of study Fees restricted to cost recovery only	Standard hospital consent

Table 3.1- continued

Resource	Number of Specimens/ Tissue Type(s)	Other Data	Limitations	Consent
National Surgical Adjuvant Breast and Bowel Project (NSABP) 320 East North Ave. Pittsburgh, PA 15212 Ph. 412-359-5013 Fax: 412-359-8685	10,000 specimens of malignant tissue from breast cancer patients enrolled in NSABP clinical trials Paraffin-embedded malignant tissue	Demographic Clinical Outcome	Available only for confirmatory studies for potential therapeutic response variables; use limited to nongenetic studies only, otherwise collaboration is required	Old tissue banks have no research-related consent. Newer protocols have consent regarding research
NCI Cooperative Breast Cancer Tissue Resource (CBCTR) Information Management Systems, Inc. 12501 Prosperity Drive, Suite 200 Silver Spring, MD 20904 Ph. 301-680-9770 Fax: 301-680-8304	8,289 primary breast cancer tissues Formalin-fixed, paraffin-embedded primary breast cancer tissues	Demographic Clinical Outcome Other	Must document IRB approval for use of human subjects; scientific merit will be determined by Research Evaluation Panel Charge for preparation of section and shipping costs	Standard hospital consent
NCI Cooperative Human Tissue Network (CHTN) (See Web site for contact information of division most relevant to research)	Specimens collected to meet researcher requests; only rare specimens banked to meet future requests Neoplastic and associated normal tissue, blood, and body fluids from routine resections and autopsies	Demographic Clinical Outcome	Cannot be used to produce commercial products. Must have evidence of IRB approval, and nominal processing fee for each specimen and shipping and handling fees	Standard hospital consent

Table 3.1- continued

Resource	Number of Specimens/ Tissue Type(s)	Other Data	Limitations	Consent
NCI Surveillance, Epidemiology, and End Results Program (SEER) 6130 Executive Blvd., Room 343J Rockville, MD 20892 Ph. 301-496-8510 Fax: 301-496-9949	Not applicable; this is a source of breast cancer-related data, not actual specimens. Database contains information on 1.7 million cancers diagnosed between 1973 and 1991; ~12,000 new cases per year	Demographic Clinical Outcome	Must not make primary data available to anyone who has not signed a confidentiality statement	Not applicable—data are unidentified and collected under state regulations
New York University Medical Center Tisch Hospital, NYU Medical Center 560 First Ave., TH466 New York, NY 10016 Ph. 212-263-8826 Fax: 212-263-7916	300 malignant samples 500 benign and precancerous samples (10 slides per case) 500 serum and blood samples Blood or blood products Frozen and paraffin-embedded malignant, benign, and normal tissue	Demographic Clinical	Fees will be levied	Standard hospital consent
North Central Cancer Treatment Group Research Base at Mayo Clinic Mayo Clinic 200 First St., S.W. Rochester, MN 55905 Ph. 507-284-4849 Fax: 507-284-1803	800 specimens from breast cancer patients entered in clinical trials over the past 10 years Paraffin-embedded malignant tissue	Demographic Clinical Outcome	Peer reviewed, scientifically meritorious uses only, and collaboration is required	Specific patient consent form is signed

Table 3.1- continued

Resource	Number of Specimens/Tissue Type(s)	Other Data	Limitations	Consent
University of Michigan Breast Cell/Tissue Bank Data and Data Base Dept. of Radiation Oncology University of Michigan Medical School 1331 East Ann St. Ann Arbor, MI 48109 Ph. 313-647-1008 Fax: 313-763-1581	Malignant: 5–10 fresh/month, >100 frozen, several hundred paraffin-embedded Normal: 1–2 fresh/month, ~20 frozen, >100 paraffin-embedded Fresh, frozen, and paraffin-embedded normal and malignant tissue Blood or blood products Cells and cell lines	Demographic Clinical Outcome	None specified	Standard hospital consent
University of Pennsylvania 1009 BRBI, 422 Currie Blvd. University of Pennsylvania Philadelphia, PA 19104 Ph. 215-898-0247 Fax: 215-662-7617	Frozen: 200 malignant, 30 benign, and 100 normal Paraffin-embedded: >1,000 malignant, >1,000 benign, >1,000 normal >500 lymphoblastoid cell lines Fresh, frozen, and paraffin-embedded normal, benign and malignant tissue Blood or blood products Lymphoblastoid cell lines	Demographic Clinical Outcome	Results reported back for inclusion in University of Pennsylvania database, and collaboration is required	Standard hospital consent for tumor tissue. Specific patient consent for immortalized cells

the 14 banks accrue as many as 200 new cases per year. A specimen from a single case can generate several samples. For example, a specimen from a single case might be split into 3–30 paraffin-embedded blocks, 10 slides, or matched frozen and paraffin-embedded tissue blocks (i.e., one frozen and one paraffin-embedded sample from the same case). Conservatively, a total of approximately 240,000 samples are included in the repositories listed in the database. Samples available to the research and clinical communities include breast tissue, serum, urine, cells, and DNA from patients diagnosed with breast cancer, those at high risk, and unaffected individuals. Information on demographics (age, sex, race, ethnicity, family history of cancer), clinical findings (pathologic diagnosis, stage, initial therapy), and outcome (subsequent breast cancer, vital status) is also available from some institutions.

NCI Cooperative Breast Cancer Tissue Resource. The Cooperative Breast Cancer Tissue Resource (CBCTR), supported by the NCI, provides access to more than 8,200 cases of formalin-fixed, paraffin-embedded primary breast cancer tissues. The current specimens represent cases accessioned from 1974 through the present. Each case receives a unique identifier. Since the block is currently part of the pathology archives, a link is kept at the collecting institution. The link provides a one-way flow of information for research purposes but is not part of the research database. Associated pathology and clinical data, such as demographic data, diagnosis, extent of disease, treatment, follow-up, recurrence, survival, and vital status, are available. However, patient identification or information about other family members will not be provided. Cases representing all stages of disease from both sexes, all ages, and all races/ethnicities are available for study. Four collaborating institutions contribute tissue and data from patients treated at their hospitals: Fox Chase Cancer Center (Fox Chase Breast Cancer Tissue Registry), Philadelphia, Pennsylvania; Kaiser Foundation Research Institute, Portland, Oregon; University of Miami, Miami, Florida; and Washington University, St. Louis, Missouri. The resource was designed for large studies to validate promising diagnostic and prognostic markers for breast cancer.

Cooperative Central Nervous System Consortium Tissue Bank. The Central Nervous System Consortium (CNSC) is funded by the Cancer Therapy Evaluation Program and the Radiation Research Program of the Division of Cancer Treatment Diagnosis and Centers at the NCI. The CNSC conducts laboratory and clinical phase I and phase II research trials to study central nervous system (CNS) tumor biology and to discover new treatments for adult patients with malignant brain tumors. The Cooperative CNSC Tissue Bank provides the consortium with a mechanism for sharing human brain tumor specimens among investigators conducting research on the biology, clinical behavior, or therapy of CNS tumors.

Biologic Specimen Bank for Early Lung Cancer Markers in Chinese Tin Miners. The Biologic Specimen Bank for Early Lung Cancer Markers in Chinese Tin Miners is maintained by the Division of Cancer Prevention and Control. The specimen bank aims to collect specimens and data that can be used for validation and refinement of potential early markers of lung cancer and to establish a cohort for the study of environmental and genetic risk factors for lung cancer. Early detection and identification and alteration of etiologic factors may reduce the incidence and mortality of lung cancer. More than 7,000 miners in the Yunnan Tin Corporation (40 years of age with 10-plus years of underground and/or smelting experience) have been enrolled in an annual lung cancer screening program for the past 20 years. Since 1992, sputum samples have been collected and stored annually for future projects on early marker identification.

NCI AIDS Malignancy Bank. The NCI AIDS Malignancy Bank (AMB), established by the NCI in 1994, consists of five "banks" located in San Francisco, Washington, D.C., Ohio, New York, and Los Angeles. Each "bank" is actually a multi-institutional consortium. The San Francisco consortium is centered at the University of California at San Francisco, coordinated by the AIDS Immunobiology Research Laboratory at San Francisco General Hospital, and consists of investigators at the major hospitals in San Francisco, New England Deaconess Medical Center in Boston, Memorial Sloan-Kettering Hospital in New York, and the Duke University Oncology Consortium of eight hospitals in the southeastern United States. The Washington, D.C., bank is a consortium operated by the Department of Pathology at George Washington University Medical Center with participation by Children's National Medical Center, Fairfax Hospital, Howard University Hospital, University of Miami, Veterans Affairs Medical Center, and Washington Hospital Center. The Ohio State AIDS Malignancy Bank is in consortium with the University of Texas Southwestern Medical Center in Dallas, Texas. The participating institutions in New York are the State University of New York Health Science Center at Brooklyn, King's County Hospital Center, and Woodhull Medical and Mental Health Center. The University of California at Los Angeles AIDS Malignancy Bank consortium includes the University of Southern California.

The AMB is a collection of tissues and biological fluids with an associated clinical database from patients with HIV-related malignancies. Currently, the AMB contains more than 18,000 samples from 2,002 cases of HIV-related malignancies. The AMB contains formalin-fixed paraffin-embedded tissues, fresh frozen tissues, malignant cell suspensions, fine needle aspirates, and cell lines from patients with HIV-related malignancies. The bank also contains serum, plasma, urine, bone marrow, cervical and anal specimens, saliva, semen, and multisite autopsy tissues from patients with HIV-related malignancies, including those who have participated in clinical trials. The bank has an associated database that contains prognostic, staging, outcome, and treatment data on patients from whom tissues were obtained. Follow-up clinical information will be requested every six months. The specimens and clinical data are available to qualified investigators in the United States for research studies, particularly those that translate basic research findings to clinical applications. Access to these specimens should encourage and facilitate research in HIV-related malignancies.

National Institute of Allergy and Infectious Disease

The National Institute of Allergy and Infectious Disease (NIAID) provides major support for scientists conducting research on improving diagnosis, prevention, and treatment of many infectious, immunologic, and allergic diseases affecting people worldwide. NIAID is composed of four extramural divisions: the Division of AIDS; the Division of Allergy, Immunology, and Transplantation; the Division of Microbiology and Infectious Disease; and the Division of Extramural Activities. Major areas of investigation include AIDS, asthma and allergic diseases, enteric diseases, malaria and other tropical diseases, and vaccine development.

The NIH AIDS Research and Reference Reagent Program (AIDS Reagent Program), established by the NIAID in 1988, is a unique resource. The AIDS Reagent Program is an AIDS Collaborating Center of the World Health Organization. It acquires critically needed reagents for AIDS-related research and provides these reagents free of charge to qualified investigators worldwide. The program contains samples of cell lines, HIV and related viruses, opportunistic infectious agents associated with HIV infections, DNA libraries, DNA clones, antibodies, purified proteins, synthetic peptides, body fluids, and reference standards.

The AIDS Reagent Program encourages collaborative research aimed at standardizing reagents and laboratory techniques. Most of the reagents are used by and donated by scientists from the NIH, academic and nonprofit institutions, and the private sector. Any commercial use of reagents requires written permission and compensation of reagent donor(s) and notification of the AIDS Reagent Program. Currently, the program has 500 registered users of its services. During the past five years the AIDS Reagent Program has provided more than 17,000 reagents to AIDS investigators worldwide.

DAIDS Specimen Repositories. The Division of the Acquired Immunodeficiency Syndrome (DAIDS) within the NIAID was established in 1986 to address the national research needs created by the HIV/AIDS epidemic. The mission of DAIDS is to increase basic knowledge of the pathogenesis, natural history, and transmission of HIV disease and to promote progress in its detection, treatment, and prevention. DAIDS supports several multi-institutional programs in epidemiologic, therapeutic, and vaccine/prevention research. Collectively, these studies have amassed a large amount of clinical data and biological specimens. The specific fluids and tissues collected vary according to study group but include peripheral blood mononuclear cells, serum, plasma, semen, saliva, vaginal washings, urine, placenta, and autopsy samples. The clinical trial studies are described below and the longitudinal studies are described in Chapter Four.

HIV Network for Prevention Trials. The HIVNET efficacy trials network is a network of clinical programs established in 1994. The mission of the HIVNET network is to conduct HIV vaccine efficacy trials and prevention trials in higher-risk populations. One of the objectives of HIVNET is to determine the incidence of HIV in higher-risk populations who may serve as good study groups for future trials.

HIVNET consists of five contracts supported by DAIDS:

1. The domestic HIV/AIDS vaccine efficacy trials master contract, which evaluates the efficacy of candidate vaccines in U.S. population.

2. The international HIV/AIDS vaccine efficacy trials master contract, which supports HIV vaccine trials in international populations.

3. The statistical and data coordinating center contract, which provides statistical and data management service for both U.S. and international trials.

4. The laboratory contract for HIV/AIDS vaccine efficacy trials, which provides specialized laboratory testing.

5. The specimen repository, which collects and archives specimens from U.S. and international trials.

The HIVNET specimen repository includes serum, plasma, peripheral mononuclear cells, genital tract secretions, and saliva. HIV strains isolated from these specimens are also available. Specimens collected from individual clinical trials are routinely sent to a central laboratory for testing. The availability of specimens depends on the type requested. Peripheral mononuclear cells are potentially available for use by collaborating investigators. Fresh specimens, such as blood or mucosal specimens, are potentially available, provided that the research offers a unique or immunological/virological assessment.

Pediatric AIDS Clinical Trials Group. The Pediatric AIDS Clinical Trials Group (PACTG) is a multicenter national clinical trials network. It supports the development and implementation of phase I, II, and III studies designed to test and optimize therapies to prevent and treat HIV infection in infants, children, and adolescents; conducts studies throughout the United States; and collaborates closely with the adult clinical trials groups, the FDA, pharmaceutical and biotechnology companies, and community constituencies to promote HIV/AIDS research.

Specimens collected from the PACTG trials include serum, plasma, peripheral mononuclear cells, culture supernatants, lymph node biopsies, tissues, urine, and other body fluids. Specimens are normally collected several times during a clinical trial. Specimens are usually sent to a specific laboratory for processing, testing, and storing. Stored specimens fall into one of two categories: protocol-specified batch testing and unspecified future studies. Specimens collected for protocol-specified batch testing are stored pending collection of all protocol specimens, at which time they undergo a protocol-specified test. Batch testing is more economical and feasible compared to "real-time" testing. Batch testing specimens are rarely available for other purposes. Specimens collected for unspecified future studies are additional specimens drawn and stored for future research.

Adult AIDS Clinical Trials Group. The Adult AIDS Clinical Trials Group (ACTG) is a consortium of 30 clinical research institutions. It conducts all phases of clinical trials designed to assess the safety and efficacy of new and improved therapies for HIV/AIDS and its associated illnesses. To date, ACTG has implemented more than 280 clinical investigations, enrolling more than 35,000 adult volunteers who are at all stages of the disease.

The goals of the ACTG are to evaluate innovative therapeutic strategies and interventions to control HIV infection; to facilitate rapid translation of basic research into clinical research and practice; and to provide a flexible resource for multidisciplinary, multicenter, clinical trials.

ACTG specimens are collected and stored several times during a clinical trial. Specimens are usually forwarded to a specific laboratory for testing. Specimens collected include serum, plasma, peripheral blood mononuclear cells, culture supernatants, lymph node biopsies, tissues, urine, and other body fluids. Specimens fall into two categories: protocol-specified batch testing and unspecified future studies, as described above for PACTG specimens.

AIDS Vaccine Evaluation Group. The AIDS Vaccine Evaluation Group (AVEG) evaluates candidate AIDS vaccines in phase I and II clinical trials for safety and immunogenicity. AVEG consists of six AIDS Vaccine Evaluation Units (AVEUs), a Statistical Coordinating Center, and a Central Immunology Laboratory. Specimens collected from AVEG studies include serum, plasma, peripheral mononuclear cells, genital tract secretions, saliva, and tears. Specimens are routinely sent to two laboratories for testing. The availability of specimens depends on the type requested. Serum specimens are usually available from all volunteers and trials. Peripheral blood mononuclear cells are potentially available for use by collaborating investigators.

Division of AIDS Treatment Research Initiative. The Division of AIDS Treatment Research Initiative (DATRI) was established to conduct phase I and II studies for HIV and associated diseases. DATRI performs small focused studies and substudies of protocols conducted by other extramural programs. DATRI clinical specimens vary according to the study under which they were collected. Many studies intentionally set aside specimens for future investigations. Samples include serum, plasma, cells and cultured cells, and supernatant from peripheral blood mononuclear cells and plasma HIV cultures.

National Heart, Lung, and Blood Institute

The Transfusion Medicine Branch of the National Heart, Lung, and Blood Institute (NHLBI) has a Blood Specimen Repository available for use by researchers for studies related to transfusion-transmitted diseases, other blood disorders, or diseases of the cardiovascular system. The repository is operated by McKesson BioServices Corp. in Maryland through an extramural contract with NHLBI. The repository, established in 1974, contains approximately 1.5 million well-characterized specimens of serum, plasma, and cells from NHLBI-sponsored studies. Since 1991, the Blood Specimen Repository has been storing an average of approximately 300,000 samples per year (see Figure 3.1) (National Heart, Lung, and Blood Institute, 1996). In 1995, the demand for specimens greatly increased. From 1991 to 1993, approximately 1,000 specimens per year were distributed to researchers, and in 1994 approximately 4,000 specimens were distributed, while in 1995, approximately 20,000 specimens were distributed (see Figure 3.2) (National Heart, Lung, and Blood Institute, 1996).

National Institute of Mental Health

The National Institute of Mental Health was originally established in 1949, left NIH and became a separate bureau with the Public Health Service in 1967, and rejoined NIH in 1992, where it is currently located. NIMH has established four major research priorities: (1) fundamental research on brain, behavior, and genetics, (2) rapid turnover of basic discoveries into research on mental disorders, (3) research that directly impacts the "real world" settings, and (4) research on child development and childhood mental disorders.

NIMH has awarded funds to three universities, the University of Alabama at Birmingham, Harvard Medical School, and Johns Hopkins University, to estab-

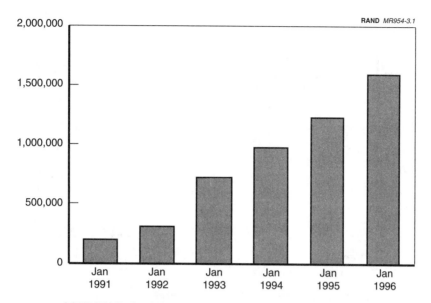

SOURCE: National Heart, Lung, and Blood Institute, Blood Specimen Repository: 1996 Catalog.

**Figure 3.1- Number of Vials Stored at the NHLBI
Blood Specimen Repository**

lish a national resource to study both early and late-onset Alzheimer's disease. A collection of samples from 400 pairs of relatives, primarily sibling pairs, are available for finding susceptibility genes linked to Alzheimer's disease. This resource provides a large enough sample of families, obtained through a common protocol and diagnosed by a consensus procedure, to be useful for identifying clinical and genetic subtypes of Alzheimer's disease.

NIMH maintains a brain collection of more than 1,200 frozen or formalin-fixed brain specimens. Brain specimens are collected from cases of schizophrenia, bipolar disorder, depression, alcoholism, drug addiction, suicides, and other cases, including AIDS, Alzheimer's, and Parkinson's disease.

National NeuroAIDS Tissue Consortium. The National NeuroAIDS Tissue Consortium (NNTC) was established in 1998 and is jointly supported by three institutes: the National Institute on Drug Abuse (NIDA), NIMH, and the National Institute of Neurological Disorders and Stroke (NINDS). The goal of the NNTC is to provide high-quality, well-characterized tissue samples to increase research efforts on HIV infection in the human brain. Four centers currently participate in the NNTC and are described below. Tissue samples will be collected from a diverse population of HIV-infected individuals and will be

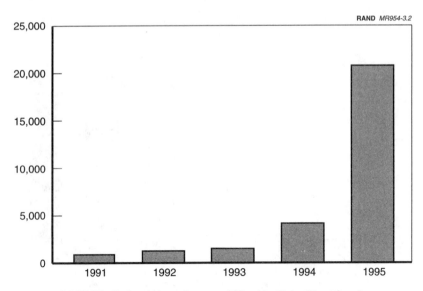

SOURCE: National Heart, Lung, and Blood Institute, Blood Specimen Repository: 1996 Catalog.

Figure 3.2- Number of Vials Distributed from the NHLBI Blood Specimen Repository

available for multiple studies. Detailed data at autopsy will be collected with all specimens, including drug use history, psychological evaluations, and clinical tests and treatment.

Mount Sinai Medical Center, New York. The Manhattan HIV Brain Bank located at the Mount Sinai Medical Center (MSSM) collects patient tissues from MSSM, Beth Israel Medical Center, and St. Luke's–Roosevelt Hospital Center in New York City. The objectives of the Manhattan HIV Brain Bank will be to identify and follow a cohort of advanced HIV patients, establish a multi-institutional clinical database, and obtain CNS, peripheral nervous system (PNS), and systemic tissues from autopsies of HIV patients; dissect, store, catalog, and distribute tissue specimens to approved investigators; and utilize pathology specimens and clinical databases in correlational studies to elucidate the pathogenesis and natural history of HIV-related neurologic diseases.

National Neurological AIDS Bank, California. The National Neurological AIDS Bank (NNAB) at UCLA will collect and store pre- and postmortem clinical data and neural tissues from autopsies for future distribution to investigators. The NNAB will also set up an electronic database and an Internet-based applications process so investigators may gain access to the bank's resources. There is no cost for the use of tissue specimens for approved investigators. The bank currently has three brains/spinal cords and 25 CSF samples.

California NeuroAIDS Tissue Network. The objective of the California Neuro-AIDS Tissue Network (CNTN) is to establish a tissue bank of CNS autopsy specimens from HIV-infected individuals who have been well-characterized neuropsychologically and neuromedically within six months of death. The CNTN represents a collaborative effort between the NIMH-funded HIV Neuro-behavioral Research Center in San Diego and four California HIV network sites: University of Southern California, Cedars-Sinai/UCLA, University of California, Irvine, and the University of California, San Diego. Collectively, these sites follow more than 4,300 patients. The CNTN seeks to identify and characterize HIV-infected persons neuromedically and neurobehaviorally following a standardized protocol, to characterize neuropathologic changes associated with HIV, to establish a tissue registry, repository, and database that can support current and future studies integrating ante- and postmortem data, and to obtain control tissue specimens. By 2003, the CNTN proposes to collect 209 sets of brain and other tissues from HIV-infected individuals with detailed ante-mortem clinical data. Seventy-five control brains from immunosuppressed patients dying after transplantation or from trauma will also be collected and stored.

Texas Repository for AIDS Neuropathogenesis Research. The Texas Repository for AIDS Neuropathogenesis Research will be based at the University of Texas Medical Branch in Galveston. The goal of the research is to establish a Texas regional brain repository to elucidate the mechanisms underlying neuro-psychological problems in AIDS patients. Frozen human brain specimens will be collected from community-based clinics in Galveston, Dallas, and Houston. Clinics in these three cities are collectively following more than 10,000 HIV-infected subjects. The brain repository will build on a prior AIDS brain repository that has almost 500 brain specimens already stored. A secure database will be established containing neuropsychiatric data, substance abuse histories, and other clinical and laboratory information.

National Institute on Aging

The National Institute on Aging (NIA) supports research on the general biology of aging and age-associated diseases and disabilities. The specific areas of research on the general biology of aging include the characterization of normal aging, cell cycle regulation and programmed cell death, stress response, and DNA damage and repair. Age-associated disease and disabilities research include the study of Alzheimer's disease, cancer, cardiovascular disease and hypertension, diabetes, and osteoporosis, osteoarthritis, and frailty. The NIA also supports the development of different intervention strategies to treat many of these age-associated diseases, such as pharmacotherapy, gene therapy, and behavioral or lifestyle changes. To provide appropriate tissue for neuro-pathological studies in Alzheimer's disease, the NIA maintains a Brain Bank.

As part of the NIA Research Resources Branch, the Central Laboratory Services Section (CLSS) collects, analyzes, and prepares for long-term storage blood and tissue samples. Other services provided by CLSS include phlebotomy, tissue handling and preservation, DNA extraction, cell transformations to create renewable cell lines, and inventory management of stored samples.

Alzheimer's Disease Research Centers. NIA funds 27 national Alzheimer's Disease Research Centers (ADRC), some of which maintain brain tissue banks described below. The ADRCs are designed to serve as shared resources to facilitate research in Alzheimer's disease. There are 14 ADRCs and 13 Alzheimer's Disease Core Centers (ADCCs). These centers provide core resources that enhance ongoing research by bringing together biomedical, behavioral, and clinical science investigators in a single center. Many of the centers provide well-characterized patients, patient and family information, and tissue and other biological samples from persons with Alzheimer's disease and from age-matched control subjects for research projects.

Kathleen Price Bryan Brain Bank. The Kathleen Price Bryan Brain Bank (Brain Bank), sponsored by NIA since 1985, is within the Alzheimer's Disease Research Center at Duke University. The major function of the Brain Bank is to retrieve and evaluate tissue for the presence of Alzheimer's neuropathologic changes and to select and retrieve human brain tissue, which will be used for further scientific investigations. The Brain Bank currently stores about 600 brains from Alzheimer's patients or related causes of dementia and 150 brains from patients with other neurological disorders, such as amyotrophic lateral sclerosis (ALS), Huntington's disease, and muscular dystrophy. The Brain Bank also has 150 brains donated from normal individuals. Fixed or frozen hemispheres, paraffin blocks, and histological slides are distributed for research, and clinical information is available.

The Taub Center for Alzheimer's Disease Research Tissue Bank. The Taub Center for Alzheimer's Disease Research Tissue Bank at Columbia-Presbyterian Medical Center is operated by the Neuropathology Core and funded by the NIA. The Tissue Bank contains flash frozen and fixed brain tissue with neurodegenerative disorders as well as normal specimens. The bank has about 300 brains stored, including those with Alzheimer's disease, Parkinson's disease, diffuse Lewy body diseases, progressive supranuclear palsy, cortico-basal ganglionic degeneration, ALS, and Creutzfeldt-Jakob disease (CJD). The bank also has peripheral blood cells and DNA stored from patients with these disorders.

Washington University Alzheimer Disease Research Center. The Washington University Alzheimer Disease Research Center (funded by NIA) has a tissue bank that is operated by the Neuropathology Core. The tissue bank collects, stores and distributes human brains, cerebrospinal fluid (CSF), and blood samples to investigators. CSF samples, heart blood samples, brain slices, and dissected anatomical regions are obtained from autopsies and stored at –80°C.

Boston University's Alzheimer's Disease Core Center. Boston University's Alzheimer's Disease Core Center operates a Brain Tissue Resource Center that supplies tissue for ongoing research projects whose focus is on any aspect of neurodegenerative diseases, especially Alzheimer's disease. The center is supported by NIA. Flash frozen and PLP immersion-fixed tissue is available from all areas of the cerebral cortex and brainstem. Brain endothelium cell cultures created from rapid postmortem samples are also available.

Michigan's Alzheimer's Disease Research Center Brain Bank. The University of Michigan Alzheimer's Disease Research Center Brain Bank was established in 1989 and its goal is to further research on Alzheimer's disease and related disorders. It is supported by NIA. The Neuropathology Core is responsible for the collection of postmortem material, part of which is frozen and part of which is used for diagnosis. Currently, more than 300 brains are stored in the Brain Bank and are available to qualified investigators nationwide.

Alzheimer's Disease Research Center at Baylor College of Medicine. The Alzheimer's Disease Research Center (ADRC) at Baylor College of Medicine was established to conduct clinical and basic science research and to diagnose and treat patients with Alzheimer's disease and related disorders. The ADRC is funded by NIA. The goal of the ADRC is to help patients, family members, and professionals cope with Alzheimer's disease through research, patient care, and education. The ADRC's research efforts target progressive deterioration of nerve cells in Alzheimer's, exploration of the potential involvement of the immune system in Alzheimer's, and mechanisms by which the beta-amyloid protein contributes to brain cell death. The ADRC maintains a serum bank of stored blood samples donated by patients who have Alzheimer's disease as well as by spouses and normal control subjects. A Brain Donation Program for Alzheimer's Disease has also been established for the collection of brain specimens for research.

The University of Kansas Medical Center Alzheimer's Disease Center. The University of Kansas Medical Center Alzheimer's Disease Center (ADC) mission is to broaden research and understanding of Alzheimer's disease and other memory disorders. The main focus of the University of Kansas Medical Center's ADC is on Alzheimer's disease and Parkinson's disease, and it is supported by NIA. The ADC has four main areas of focus: a clinical program, a brain bank, an educational program, and a research program. The clinical program has developed and maintains a large database registry of Alzheimer's disease, Parkinson's disease, and normal control subjects for research studies. The neuropathology core has established a brain bank to collect brain tissue from normal control subjects and persons with Alzheimer's and Parkinson's disease for research studies. The brain bank serves as a repository of nervous system tissue that allows for the correlation of clinical and neuropathological findings. The education program provides information about Alzheimer's and Parkinson's disease to professionals, patients, families, and the general public. A major goal of the ADC research program is the development of effective pharmacotherapy for Alzheimer's and Parkinson's disease.

University of California, Los Angeles (UCLA), Alzheimer's Disease Center. The UCLA Alzheimer's Disease Center (ADC) consists of five cores: administrative, clinical (including six clinical sites), imaging, pathology, and education/information transfer. The center is supported by NIA. The UCLA ADC has also established a brain bank. More than 800 patients and controls have been evaluated by the Clinical Core or are linked into the Clinical Core database, 639 structural and functional images have been obtained through the Imaging Core, and more than 100 brains have been examined in the Pathology Core.

Rush Alzheimer's Disease Center. The Alzheimer's Disease Center at Rush-Presbyterian–St. Luke's Medical Center focuses on four main areas of research: identifying risk factors for Alzheimer's disease, understanding the presentation and course of Alzheimer's disease, investigating underlying neurobiologic causes of Alzheimer's disease, and developing treatments for Alzheimer's disease. The Rush Center is supported by NIA. The Rush Alzheimer's Disease Center Brain Bank has two objectives: to provide neuropathological diagnosis of Alzheimer's disease by postmortem evaluation and to facilitate research of the etiology of Alzheimer's disease. More than 1,000 brain autopsies have been conducted by the brain bank since 1987. Cerebrospinal fluid samples, serum, DNA, and white blood cells are also collected by the brain bank. All tissue specimens are available to outside investigators throughout the United States.

Indiana Alzheimer Disease Center. The Indiana Alzheimer Disease Center (ADC) comprises six cores and is supported by NIA. The Indiana ADC has focused its studies on AD patients within the African-American community, on clinical and neuropathologic studies of familial forms of AD and other hereditary degenerative adult onset dementias, on trials for new drug therapies for AD, and on educational activities.

The Indiana ADC maintains a National Cell Repository that has collected genetic material from more than 2,200 individuals from 440 families with histories of AD. Both lymphocytes and DNA are available from most participants.

Family pedigrees are available for participating AD families. Tissues from various types of AD families are stored in the repository, including families with autopsy-confirmed cases of AD, families with multiple affected siblings, two-generation affected families, and early and late-onset AD families. Cell lines and DNA are available to approved investigators at no cost.

Northwestern University's Alzheimer's Disease Core Center. The goal of the Alzheimer's Disease Core Center (ADCC) at Northwestern University is to establish a clinical registry of well-characterized patients with Alzheimer's disease and other dementias and healthy elderly subjects. The center is supported by NIA. The ADCC will focus on basic mechanisms of the disease, clinical symptoms, treatments, and caregiving aspects. A brain endowment program has been established to collect normal and diseased brain tissue for research.

University of Rochester Alzheimer's Disease Center. The Alzheimer's Disease Center (ADC) at the University of Rochester consists of four cores: administrative, clinical (including two satellite diagnostic centers), neuropathology (brain bank), and education and information transfer. The center is supported by NIA. The ADC is designed to serve a broad range of studies, particularly in the area of clinical studies and trials of therapeutic interventions. Neuropathologic examination of brains has been expanded to distinguish Lewy bodies and plaque subtypes.

Emory University's Alzheimer's Disease Center. The Alzheimer's Disease Center (ADC) was established in 1991 at Emory University and is supported by NIA. The ADC consists of five cores: administrative and data management, clinical, neuropathology, molecular biology, and education and transfer. The Clinical Core examines a high proportion of African-American subjects and provides research, clinical, and educational opportunities to the African-American community. The Neuropathology Core supplies brain and other tissues from its brain bank of cases of well-characterized dementia and control cases to investigators.

University of Washington Alzheimer's Disease Research Center. The Alzheimer's Disease Research Center (ADRC) at the University of Washington focuses on understanding the basic mechanisms underlying the development of adult dementing disorders, specifically on susceptibility factors underlying Alzheimer's disease. The ADRC consists of five major research projects and seven supporting core units, including a cell tissue and fluid bank. The center is supported by NIA. A Clinical Registry Core has been established at a satellite site devoted to underserved populations in the region.

The ADRC Core, Cell, Tissue and Fluid Bank Cell Culture and Cytogenetics is one of the oldest repositories for familial AD pedigrees. The core maintains AD and control lymphoblastoid cell lines, fibroblasts, lymphocytes, and plasma.

Tissue specimens are available to ADRC investigators and approved investigators at the University of Washington and other institutions.

University of California, Davis, Alzheimer's Disease Center. The objectives of the Alzheimer's Disease Center (ADC) at the University of California, Davis, are to educate health professionals and the public about Alzheimer's disease and related dementias, to conduct research in clinical and community populations into the causes and potential treatments for dementia, and to advocate changes in health policy and practice that will enhance the recognition, treatment, and management of dementia. The center is supported by NIA. Research studies are focused on the behavioral and mental changes of dementing disorders, genetics of Alzheimer's disease, and strategies to prevent mental loss.

The Neuropathology Core at the UC Davis ADC has three major goals: to obtain brain autopsies on ADC patients and controls, to accurately diagnose brain lesions encountered at autopsy, and to preserve and distribute autopsy brain tissues to research collaborators. Brains are removed within 24 hours of death and half the brain is formalin-fixed and the other half is coronally sectioned and frozen. Twenty-five blocks of the formalin-fixed tissue are obtained for paraffin embedment from multiple neocortical, limbic, diencephalic, basal ganglia, and brainstem regions. A standard gross and microscopic neuropathology examination is performed on each new brain specimen. An inventory of all tissue specimens, the mode of processing and storage, pathological diagnosis, and autolysis interval are maintained in a neuropathology laboratory database.

Case Western Reserve Alzheimer Center. The Alzheimer Center at Case Western Reserve University consists of seven departments and is supported by NIA. Research projects include studies on apolipoprotein E, brain electrical studies of attention in Alzheimer's disease, clinical studies to design effective treatments for Alzheimer's disease, life history studies, changes in emotional responsivity studies, and visual spatial studies. The Neuropathology Core provides adequately preserved and well-characterized human brain tissue samples for biochemical and morphometric studies. The core has examined and stored 183 brains, 123 of which were diagnosed with pure Alzheimer's disease or in combination with other processes. The core has also examined and stored 554 brains, 397 of which with prion diseases.

National Institute on Deafness and Other Communication Disorders

The National Institute on Deafness and Other Communication Disorders (NIDCD) was established in 1988, splitting off from the National Institute of Neurological and Communicative Disorders and Stroke. NIDCD conducts and supports biomedical and behavioral research and research training in the normal and disordered processes of hearing, balance, smell, taste, voice, speech, and language. NIDCD also conducts and supports research and research training related to disease prevention and health promotion and addresses special biomedical and behavioral problems associated with people who have communication impairments or disorders.

NIDCD established the National Temporal Bone, Hearing and Balance Pathology Resource Registry in 1992. The registry was originally founded as the National Temporal Bone Banks Program (NTBB) in 1960 by the Deafness Research Foundation (DRF) to encourage individuals with ear disorders to donate their temporal bones at death for scientific research. The NTBB, however, became virtually inactive in the 1980s due to rising costs, dwindling funds, and a decrease of investigations in the area of temporal bone research. In 1988, a workshop cosponsored by NIDCD and DRF reaffirmed the importance of temporal bone research and NIDCD established the new registry in 1992, which would assume the responsibilities of the NTBB.

The contract of the registry was awarded to the Massachusetts Eye and Ear Infirmary and DRF. The services and functions of the registry include establishing a computerized database of human temporal bone collections, dissemination of information about the temporal bone collections, the implementation of professional educational activities in the study of human temporal bones and auditory brain stems and the development and implementation of a national acquisition network to increase the yield of human temporal bone and brain tissue from donors.

The registry's temporal bone database contains information from more than 6,300 cases (12,000 specimens) from 18 U.S. temporal bone collections. It provides basic information on the specimens and catalogues all known processed human temporal bones and related brain tissue specimens in the United States and the data associated with these specimens, such as clinical and histopathological diagnoses.

There are 26 temporal bone laboratories in the United States that possess temporal bone collections, though only 15 actively collect, process, and study temporal bone specimens. The active laboratories are listed below and their collections are described in detail in Appendix C:

Baylor College of Medicine, Houston, Texas

Bowman-Gray School of Medicine, Winston-Salem, North Carolina

Eye and Ear Institute of Pittsburgh, Pittsburgh, Pennsylvania

Goodhill Ear Center (UCLA), Los Angeles, California

Johns Hopkins University, Baltimore, Maryland

University of Michigan, Ann Arbor, Michigan

Massachusetts Eye and Ear Infirmary, Boston, Massachusetts

Mt. Sinai School of Medicine, New York, New York

New York University Medical Center, New York, New York

SUNY Health Science Center, Syracuse, New York

University of Chicago, Chicago, Illinois

The University of Iowa Hospitals and Clinics, Iowa City, Iowa

University of Minnesota, Minneapolis, Minnesota

University of Texas Southwestern Medical Center, Dallas, Texas

National Institute of Environmental Health Sciences

The mission of the National Institute of Environmental Health Sciences (NIEHS) is to reduce the burden of human illness and dysfunction from environmental causes by understanding each of these elements and their interactions. NIEHS achieves its mission through multidisciplinary biomedical research programs and prevention and intervention efforts. One way NIEHS achieves its mission by funding environmental health centers throughout the United States. The mission of these centers is multifold and includes strengthening the research focus and accomplishments of the host institution in environmental health science; supporting core facilities, which provide access to technology that enhances the research productivity of the center; and stimulating multidisciplinary research. Institutions that have NIEHS-sponsored centers include Harvard, Oregon State, Vanderbilt, University of California at Berkeley, and MIT. Several of the centers collect and store human samples for use by the center's investigators. Four NIEHS Centers that collect and store human samples for research are described below.

Kresge Center for Environmental Health Studies. The Kresge Center for Environmental Health Studies at Harvard University was established in 1958 to promote interactions among biological scientists, physical scientists, and engineers working on environmental problems concerning human health. Six scientific cores and four facility cores provide equipment and technicians for services for center investigators. One of the facility cores is the Human Cell Bank, Genotyping, and Tissue Culture Facility. The mission of the Human Cell Bank, Genotyping, and Tissue Culture Facility is to provide resources and services for Center investigators, including the acquisition, storage, and characterization of human cells and tissues. The primary focus of the cell bank has been on diploid fibroblasts isolated from three different populations: individuals with defined syndromes, exhibiting an enhanced predisposition to cancer; families present-ing with either multiple cancers, early onset cancers, or rarer types of cancers; and cells from individuals showing unusual clinical responses to radiation or chemotherapy. Cell lines banked in the facility include human diploid fibro-blast strains, including normal cells and cells from individuals with cancer sus-ceptibility syndromes and DNA repair defects; 16 human tumor cell lines; six engineered cell lines expressing transfected genes; strains from five hereditary retinoblastoma families; 10 colorectal cancer cell lines; six glioblastoma cell lines; and 15 head and neck cancer cell lines.

Environmental Health Sciences Center. The Environmental Health Sciences Center at the University of Southern California (USC) was established in 1996. The center is a consortium of almost 50 investigators from USC, UCLA, and Caltech. The center seeks to create an interdisciplinary approach to the study and advancement of research in environmental health. The center consists of an administrative core, five research cores, and four service cores. One of the four service cores is the Biological Sampling Processing Facility Core. The mis-sion of the Biological Sampling Processing Facility Core is to provide a single center to assist researchers from about 150 clinical facilities. Services provided by the facility include development of samples handling protocols, receipt of newly collected samples, and the monitoring of the quality of incoming sam-ples. Biological samples stored at the facility include blood, tissue, urine, other body fluids, smears, and scrapings (e.g., buccal cells). Several different research studies have contributed tissue samples to the Facility Core. The Genotyping and Risk of Asthma study has collected more than 1,000 buccal scrapings from school children from various communities. The Gene-Diet/Tobacco Inter-actions in Breast Cancer in Asians has collected 500 out of an anticipated 800 frozen buffy coats (white blood cells) for study of variant alleles in detoxifying enzymes. The Determinants of Childhood Susceptibility to Air Pollution study has collected 1,000 buccal smears from school children for genotype analysis.

Center for Ecogenetics and Environmental Health. The Center for Ecogenetics and Environmental Health at the University of Washington includes seven major research cores, six facility cores, and an administration core. The objec-tives of the center are to foster interdisciplinary collaborations among researchers working in the fields of toxicology, molecular biology, genetics, and environmental epidemiology and to stimulate the transition of basic mech-anistic research on molecular biomarkers of disease susceptibility to studies in the human population. The Human Studies Facilities Core's objectives are to facilitate collaborations between investigators with expertise in human popula-tion-based studies and novel or complicated methodologies. The core has a –80°C freezer and access to a fully equipped lab for preserving tissue samples. The Human Studies Resources Facility Core has worked on establishing and promoting the use of the Registry for the Study of Genetic and Environmental Risk Factors. This registry consists of demographic data, medical history information, and DNA from blood or buccal cells. Registrants are study subjects participating in projects conducted by Center investigators.

Institute of Toxicology and Environmental Health. The Institute of Toxicology and Environmental Health at the University of California, Davis, is composed of five research cores and seven facility cores. The focus of the center's research is on agricultural chemicals and related xenobiotics. The Field Studies Facility Core provides services and consulting expertise related to agricultural epidemiologic investigations, field exposure assessments, and biostatistics. Human tissues and fluids are collected from the center's epidemiologic studies of subjects in agriculture. The Field Studies Service Core provides resources for the application of laboratory methods on agricultural workers and the collection of specimens for laboratory analysis. Specimens are analyzed for exposure and toxicological effects of agrochemicals. Specimens from workers include blood and urine samples.

National Institute of Diabetes and Digestive and Kidney Diseases

The National Institute of Diabetes and Digestive and Kidney Diseases (NIDDK) split from the National Institute of Arthritis, Diabetes, and Digestive and Kidney Diseases in 1988. NIDDK's Division of Intramural Research conducts studies on diabetes, inborn errors of metabolism, endocrine disorders, mineral metabolism, digestive diseases, nutrition, urology and kidney diseases, and hematology. Extramural research at NIDDK is separated into five divisions: Diabetes, Endocrinology and Metabolic Diseases; Digestive Diseases and Nutrition; Kidney, Urologic, and Hematologic Diseases; Extramural Activities; and Nutrition Research Coordination.

The Liver Tissue Procurement and Distribution System (LTPADS) is sponsored by NIDDK to provide human liver tissues from three regional centers in the United States for NIH investigators. These regional centers have active liver transplant programs to provide portions of resected pathologic liver. Frozen or fresh tissue is available for common forms of childhood and adult cirrhosis, fulminant liver failure, chronic rejection, and inborn errors of metabolism. Normal liver specimens may be requested, but the supply is much more limited and it usually takes much longer to fulfill requests.

NATIONAL INSTITUTE OF STANDARDS AND TECHNOLOGY AND THE U.S. ENVIRONMENTAL PROTECTION AGENCY

Two other agencies within the federal government have tissue banks: the National Institute of Standards and Technology (NIST) and the U.S. Environmental Protection Agency (EPA). These tissue banks were established primarily to determine human exposure to pollutants and pesticides and to follow long-term trends.

National Biomonitoring Specimen Bank

The National Biomonitoring Specimen Bank (NBSB) at the NIST was established in 1979 in conjunction with the EPA to determine the feasibility of long-term storage of environmental samples (Wise and Koster, 1995). In addition to the specimens contained in the human liver specimen bank supported by the EPA, the NBSB also archives specimens from three other projects supported by various government agencies, such as marine specimens and total human diet specimens. The EPA human liver specimen bank collected and archived 661 human liver specimens from 1980 through 1994 from individuals in Seattle, Baltimore, and Minneapolis. The goals of the EPA human liver project were to develop procedures for the collection, processing, and long-term storage of biologic specimens; to improve analytical methods for the determination of inorganic and organic contaminants in human tissue; to evaluate the long-term storage stability of biologic specimens; and to provide an archive of well-documented specimens of human liver for retrospective studies to determine long-term pollution trends and document the appearance of new pollutants (Wise and Koster, 1995). This archive of human liver specimens is an invaluable resource for the investigation of environmental pollution trends in human population.

National Human Monitoring Program

The National Human Monitoring Program (NHMP) was established in 1967 and continued through 1993. The NHMP was designed to study changes in pesticide residues in the population of the United States. Originally part of the U.S. Public Health Service, the NHMP was transferred to the EPA in 1970. One of the primary activities of the NHMP was the National Human Adipose Tissue Survey (NHATS), a program developed to measure residues of chemicals in human adipose tissue. Through 1991, the NHATS had collected approximately 12,000 samples of adipose tissue from autopsied cadavers and surgical patients. The NHATS documented widespread exposure to pesticides in the United States and showed that reduced use of polychlorinated biphenyls (PCBs), DDT, and dieldrin resulted in lower tissue concentrations of these compounds (Bailar, 1995).

RESEARCH UNIVERSITIES AND ACADEMIC MEDICAL CENTERS

Research universities and academic medical centers maintain formal tissue banks for distribution throughout the research community as well as core facilities to support their own research. Examples of both types of tissue collections are described below.

AIDS Specimen Bank at the University of California at San Francisco

The University of California at San Francisco (UCSF) AIDS Specimen Bank has been in existence since 1982 and has banked more than 76,000 samples and distributed more than 82,000 specimens to researchers worldwide. Specimens include serum, tissue, saliva, cells, and cerebrospinal fluid from HIV infected individuals. Specimen data are archived in a computerized database. The bank provides investigators with specimens for basic, epidemiological, and clinical research.

The Brain Bank

The Brain Bank is one of two core facilities at the Alzheimer's Research Center (ARC) at the Medical College of Georgia. The ARC was established in 1989 with start-up funds provided by the Calloway Foundation of Georgia. The goal of the ARC is to continue to help investigators, technical scientists, and graduate trainees to better understand the causes of Alzheimer's disease and to develop new treatment strategies through research. Ongoing research at the ARC primarily involves basic science aspects of Alzheimer's disease. The Brain Bank currently stores 24 brains, mostly from Alzheimer's disease patients.

Brain Bank Core

The Brain Bank Core at the Mount Sinai School of Medicine of the City University of New York will obtain, characterize, describe, dissect, preserve, and distribute brain tissues from normal controls and Alzheimer's disease subjects to different investigators involved in Alzheimer's disease research. The Brain Bank Core is supported by the NIA. The right half of the brain will be preserved in paraformaldehyde for neuropathological and neuroanatomical studies, and the left half will be dissected into coronal slabs and snap-frozen. The Brain Bank Core will serve five projects in the Department of Psychiatry: Neuropathology, Neuropsychology, Family History, Acute Phase Reactants, and Neurochemistry projects. Tissues from the Brain Bank Core will also be available for projects funded by other grants.

Brain and Tissue Bank for Developmental Disorders at the University of Maryland, Baltimore, the University of Miami, and Children's Hospital of Orange County

The Brain and Tissue Banks for Developmental Disorders at the University of Maryland, Baltimore, the University of Miami, and the Children's Hospital of Orange County, supported by the National Institute of Child Health and Human Development (NICHD), were established to advance the research of developmental and childhood disorders. The tissue banks systematically collect, store, and distribute brain and other tissues for research dedicated to improving understanding, care, and treatment of individuals with developmental disorders. The Brain and Tissue Banks store tissues, either frozen or formalin-fixed, of almost all tissue types from both normal and diseased donors. A smaller Ataxia Telangiectasia Patient Brain Tissue Bank exists as a subset of the Brain and Tissue Banks.

Breast Cancer Database and Biologic Resource Bank

The University of Washington's Breast Cancer Database and Biologic Resource Bank was established to facilitate the development of a national resource of biologic materials linked to a substantial database. A comprehensive database, tumor tissue bank, and serum/lymphocyte bank was developed from breast cancer patients at the University of Washington Medical Center. Other biological specimens may be collected from these patients, such as bone marrow, skin biopsies, lymph node biopsies, metastatic tumor samples, and benign breast tissue.

Breast Tissue Repository

The Breast Tissue Repository (BTR), at the Hamon Center for Therapeutic Oncology Research in the University of Texas Southwestern's Medical Center, was initiated in the early 1990s and is supported by a U.S. Army grant and funds from the Susan Komen Foundation. The goal of BTR is to create a comprehensive breast tissue/cell repository as a research source for investigators. The repository contains cell lines generated from breast tumor tissues and cryopreserved epithelial and stromal cell lines. Detailed information on the cellular, biochemical, and molecular analysis of these cell lines along with a comprehensive record of clinical and pathological data are available for the breast tumor cell lines.

Breast Tumor Bank

The Breast Tumor Bank at the University of California, Los Angeles, was established for use in basic molecular, biochemical, and epidemiologic studies of
human breast cancer. The tumor bank collects and archives malignant breast
tissue, premalignant breast tissue, and bone marrow and peripheral blood
samples from breast cancer patients. Relevant clinical, demographic, epidemiological, and pathologic data is collected along with each specimen. If
sufficient tissue is available, it is processed for DNA, RNA, tissue powder, and
tissue fragments (both frozen and paraffin-embedded). Tissue specimens are
available for approved studies.

Cancer Center Tissue Core at University of California, San Francisco (UCSF)

The UCSF Cancer Center is an interdisciplinary group that combines basic scientific study, clinical research, epidemiology/cancer control, and patient care
services into one program. The Cancer Center's mission is the discovery and
evolution of new ideas and information about cancer. The UCSF Cancer Center
Tissue Core is a centralized facility that identifies and stores patient tissue. The
goal of the Tissue Core is to provide specimens to approved investigators. The
Tissue Core collects fresh, frozen, and formalin-fixed, paraffin-embedded tissue
from a variety of organs, including breast, prostate, and bladder.

Cancer Tissue Bank

The VA Medical Center in Minneapolis, Minnesota, maintains a bank of frozen
cancer tissue and paired normal tissue sections for future research in onco-
genesis and outcome studies. The tissue bank is supported by the Department
of Veterans Affairs. Samples will be collected from neoplasms along with non-
cancerous samples adjacent to tumors. Clinical information, such as type of
treatment, exposure to cancer risk factors, and outcome data, can be obtained
from the Minneapolis VA Medical Center Tumor Registry or chart review. Currently, more than 2,000 tumor samples have been collected.

Cell and Tissue Bank for Marker Studies of Diseases of the Bladder, Prostate, Kidney, Lung, and Breast

The Cell and Tissue Bank for Marker Studies of Diseases of the Bladder,
Prostate, Kidney, Lung, and Breast is located at the Veterans Affairs Medical
Center in Oklahoma City, Oklahoma. The Cell and Tissue Bank is supported by
the Department of Veterans Affairs. The bank stores blood cells and bladder

washes and tissue samples from patients with diseases, including cancer of the bladder, prostate, or kidney, and blood and tissue samples of patients with such diseases as colon and breast cancer. Patient information (e.g., outcome, demographic, medical, and lifestyle information) is collected with each sample. The Cell and Tissue Bank specimens are used in studies to characterize objective biomedical markers in cells for the purpose of improving markers for disease detection, monitoring, and risk assessment.

Central Prostate Cancer Serum Repository

The NCI supports the Central Prostate Cancer Serum Repository at the VA Medical Center in Lexington, Kentucky. The objective of the repository is to establish a serum bank to collect and store serum of patients with prostate cancer entered into Southwest Oncology Group–approved studies. Serum samples will be distributed to investigators for projects on new or existing markers or other tests in a prospective or retrospective design.

Collection of DNA/RNA Tissue Repository for Neurodegenerative Disorders

The Collection of DNA/RNA Tissue Repository for Neurodegenerative Disorders is located in the Department of Neurology at Baylor College of Medicine. The aims of the DNA/RNA Bank are to establish a detailed database for patients with neurodegenerative disorders and to collect blood samples for future DNA analysis. If the disease is hereditary, family members are included in the database and blood samples are collected. Subjects are asked to provide information in a questionnaire about their symptoms and family involvement. The DNA/RNA bank is for internal use only. In addition to the blood samples collected, limited brain and muscle specimens are stored at –80°C and in liquid nitrogen, respectively. Demographic and detailed clinical data is obtained for each specimen.

DNA Bank to Detect Gene Polymorphisms in Heart Failure

The Department of Veterans Affairs supports the establishment of a large bank of genomic DNA samples derived from peripheral blood lymphocytes from patients with etiologically defined heart failure and from matched population controls. The bank is located at the VA Medical Center in Little Rock, Arkansas. These samples will be frozen and stored for future studies that analyze specific genetic loci of interest. Ethnic group and family history will be collected with each sample.

Early Detection Research Network- Tissue Bank for Matched Tissues to Screen for Markers of Neoplastic Progression

The VA Medical Center in Birmingham, Alabama, has collected a group of matched tissues from operations and preoperative body fluids to be stored in a tissue bank. The tissue bank is supported by the Department of Veterans Affairs. Specimens will include blood, urine, and feces from preoperative patients and remnant tissue sections from the surgical specimen. Patients with inflammatory diseases diagnosed or treated by surgery/biopsy will serve as controls. These specimens will be used in studies investigating whether chemicals present in the body, in tissues, or in fluids can be measured to predict the progression of tumors. Specimens will be analyzed for biomarkers that can be correlated with early detection, diagnosis, and prognosis of the patient's disease process.

Gift of Hope Brain Bank for AIDS

The Gift of Hope Brain Bank for AIDS at the VA Medical Center in Los Angeles, California, is supported by the Department of Veterans Affairs. The brain bank recruits, collects, preserves, and banks high-quality tissue and CSF/serum specimens. All specimens are quick-frozen and available at no charge to investigators for study of AIDS dementia and other AIDS-related neurologic symptoms. Medical and neuropathological records are also available to investigators.

Harvard Brain Tissue Resource Center

The Harvard Brain Tissue Resource Center (The Brain Bank), at McLean Hospital in Massachusetts, is a centralized repository for the collection and distribution of postmortem human brain specimens from both diseased and normal donors for use in research on the brain and nervous system. The Brain Bank is supported by the NIMH, the National Institutes of Neurological Disease and Stroke, the Alzheimer Disease Association of Indiana, the Hereditary Disease Foundation, the Tourette Syndrome Association, and the Wills Foundation. Research on brain tissue has contributed to the understanding of severe mental illness, the development of a genetic test for Huntington's disease, and a treatment for Parkinson's disease. The mission of the Brain Bank is to serve as a national resource for the collection and distribution of postmortem brain tissue for medical research into the causes of neurological and severe psychiatric disorders. Because the majority of research requires very small amounts of tissue, each donated brain provides a large number of samples for many researchers. Brain tissue donations are accepted by the Brain Bank from individuals or the parents, siblings, and offspring of individuals with such severe neurological disorders as Huntington's, Parkinson's, and Alzheimer's diseases, with a serious psychiatric diagnosis, and various other disorders. The Brain Bank also accepts brain tissue from normal individuals with no neurological or neuropsychiatric disorders for research that needs to compare normal tissue with diseased tissue. Prospective brain tissue donors must be 18 years of age or older. Donors should discuss their wishes with their families and can register with the Brain Bank by completing the "Brain Donation Questionnaire."

Brain tissues are stored as fresh quick-frozen tissue blocks and coronal sections, passive frozen hemispheres, and formalin-fixed hemispheres. Researchers can request custom dissection of specified anatomic regions of the passive frozen or formalin-fixed hemispheres. All tissue diagnoses are confirmed by retrospective review of clinical records and a comprehensive neuropathological examination. There is no cost for distribution of brain tissues to approved researchers.

The Harvard Psychiatry Brain Collection was created as a subsidiary of the Harvard Brain Tissue Resource Center. This collection specifically attempts to collect brain tissue from families with serious mental illness. Tissues from patients with schizophrenia, manic-depression, obsessive-compulsive disorder, and first-degree relatives of individuals with these disorders are being collected for research and distributed to qualified investigators.

HIV-Related Malignancy Tissue/Biological Fluids Bank

A consortium of Washington, D.C., metropolitan hospitals has established a comprehensive bank of biological fluids and tissue specimens from individuals with HIV-related malignancies. The HIV bank is supported by the Department of Veterans Affairs and is in the Department of Pathology at George Washington University. Diagnostic tissue (either fresh-frozen or formalin-fixed) and biological fluids (blood, urine, and other fluids) are collected from HIV seropositive individuals who have HIV-related malignancies. The specimens are available to researchers throughout the United States for approved requests.

Human Brain Bank

The Human Brain Bank Core at the University of Pittsburgh, Department of Psychiatry was established in 1990 and is supported by the NIMH. The goal of the brain bank is to identify, recover, assess, and distribute postmortem human brain specimens from cases of schizophrenia and matched normal control and nonschizophrenic psychiatric comparison subjects. Clinical features of each specimen and its availability are stored in a database and are accessible to center investigators.

Human Gastrointestinal Tumor Bank

The Human Gastrointestinal Tumor Bank was established to provide human tissue samples for the investigation of the molecular basis of carcinogenesis. The tumor bank is located at the VA Medical Center in Nashville, Tennessee, and is supported by the Department of Veterans Affairs. Tissue samples will be obtained from surgical specimens of esophageal, gastric, pancreatic, and colon carcinoma cases. Specimens are fixed or frozen. Clinical diagnoses and relevant clinical information are collected and maintained for each specimen. Current research projects utilizing these tissue samples include determination of the proliferative index by PCNA immunohistochemistry and in vitro staining and localization of the epidermal growth factor/transforming growth factor family of ligands and receptors in normal, adenomatous, and malignant tissue.

Human Lung Cancer Tissue Resource

The VA Medical Center in Albuquerque, New Mexico, has established the Human Lung Cancer Tissue Resource. The tissue resource is supported by the Department of Veterans Affairs and its objective is to collect samples of lung tumors for long-term tissue banking. The tissue resource provides specimens for investigators interested in lung carcinogenesis. Data, including exposure history and employment history, are collected from each specimen. Tumor specimens as well as normal specimens are collected. Currently, the tissue resource has collected 236 tumor samples.

Inflammatory Bowel Disease Tissue Bank

The Inflammatory Bowel Disease Tissue Bank at Massachusetts General Hospital, established in 1988, is funded by the National Institute of Diabetes and Digestive and Kidney Diseases (NIDDK). The tissue bank stores specimens from cases of Crohn's disease and ulcerative colitis, as well as colon cancer, adenocarcinoma, and diverticular disease. More than 250 cases are archived with three to five specimens from each case and data regarding final diagnosis, age, and sex of the patient are catalogued with each specimen. The specimens are available to investigators at no cost.

International Registry of Werner Syndrome/Cell Bank

The University of Washington has established the International Registry of Werner Syndrome/Cell Bank supported by the NCI. Werner syndrome is a rare disorder that causes premature aging and early death. The registry has been in existence since 1990 and has collected lymphoblastoid cell lines, primary skin fibroblasts and SV40-transformed fibroblast cultures containing a wide range of Werner syndrome mutations. A collection of sib-pairs (wild type versus hetero-zygotic carrier) will be available for retrospective and long-term prospective studies of the susceptibility of heterozygotes to various types of neoplasms. All specimens are available to investigators associated with the Program Project grant. In addition, cultures representative of a variety of mutations are avail-able to the general community.

LSU Neuroscience Center Brain Tissue Bank

The Neuroscience Center of Excellence at Louisiana State University maintains a Brain Tissue Bank. The Brain Tissue Bank obtains, processes, and distributes postmortem human brain tissue to investigators for neuroscience research.

Lung Cancer in Uranium Miners: A Tissue Resource

The VA Medical Center in Albuquerque, New Mexico, has established a tissue bank to store samples of lung cancers and other tissues of lung cancer patients. The tissue resource is supported by the Department of Veterans Affairs. Tissue samples collected from lung cancer patients include cancer, blood, and spu-tum. Currently, tissue samples from 248 patients with lung cancer have been collected.

Massachusetts General Hospital Tumor Bank

The Massachusetts General Hospital (MGH) Tumor Bank was established in 1996 as a joint effort by MGH Cancer Center, the Hematology/Oncology Divi-sion of the Department of Medicine, and the Department of Pathology. Its goal is to collect and distribute surgical specimens of human tumors for biomedical research. Tumor specimens are collected from surgeries conducted at MGH. Resected specimens are sent to the pathology lab for diagnosis and excess tis-sue is snap-frozen and stored at the Tumor Bank. Specimens are distributed to researchers for approved scientific studies.

Mental Health Clinical Research Center Brain Bank

The Mental Health Clinical Research Center Brain Bank was established to provide neuroscientists with normal and abnormal brain morphology and neurochemistry in psychiatric conditions. The brain bank at the VA Medical Center in Iowa City, Iowa, is supported by the Department of Veterans Affairs. Tissues collected include brains from normal individuals and persons suffering from major mental illness. Brain specimens are sliced coronally in the fresh state, and alternate slices are fixed or flash-frozen. Tissues are digitized to record anatomical appearances prior to storage. Tissue blocks are available to investigators for morphometric and chemical analyses.

Mucosal Immunology Core

The Mucosal Immunology Core at the University of California, Los Angeles, is supported by the National Institute of Allergy and Infectious Diseases. Mucosal lymphoid tissue has been shown to be a major reservoir of replicative HIV-1. Recent studies are investigating differential rates of CD4+ T-cell depletion in lymphoid tissue versus peripheral blood. The gut-associated lymphoid tissue is the body's major lymphoid organ and is accessible by endoscopic biopsy. The Mucosal Immunology Core provides investigators with clinically well-characterized tissue specimens from gastrointestinal mucosal sites. Fresh and frozen samples will be collected from seropositive subjects and seronegative controls. Site-specific biopsies can be obtained via request for studies requiring esophageal, stomach, duodenal, ileal, colonic, and rectal tissue. Mononuclear mucosal preparations and immunoglobulin secretions from saliva or rectal mucosa may also be collected prospectively. In addition, other mucosal tissues (pharyngeal, pulmonary, vaginal, urinary system) and samples from other patient populations (women and minorities) are available.

Neuropathology Core

A Neuropathology Core has been established in the Department of Microbiology at the University of Pennsylvania. The project was initiated in 1994 and is supported by the NINDS. The objectives of the core are to conduct histopathological-based studies to compare the cellular distribution of HIV and cytokines with pathological lesions and to establish a brain tissue bank. Brain tissues will be stored in various ways to optimize their use in other projects. About 10 brains will be collected each year.

Oral Cancer Research Center

The Oral Cancer Research Center at the University of California, San Francisco, has established a tissue and histopathology core to provide fundamental support to research investigators. The core makes available human oral cancerous and precancerous tissues for applied research studies, develops a patient database for correlation of patient outcome with molecular tumor markers, and provides basic, technical, histologic, and immunohistologic services to center investigators. Tissue will be collected from new patients treated at UCSF clinical sites and from pathology archives of five UCSF hospitals and two large San

Francisco oral pathology biopsy services. Biopsies and surgical specimens with a diagnosis of oral epithelial dysplasia, carcinoma in situ, invasive carcinoma, and verrucal carcinoma will also be collected.

A secondary source of tissue will be five additional California oral pathology services and two west coast oral medicine clinics. More than 3,000 archived oral cancers and precancers are immediately available for study, and an estimated 125 new tumors will be accessioned annually from the San Francisco Bay area for use in prospective studies.

Prediagnostic Breast Cancer Serum Bank

The Prediagnostic Breast Cancer Serum Bank was created as part of the Biological Markers Project at the NCI. Between 1977 and 1987, blood from more than 7,300 women free of breast cancer was collected. The Division of Cancer Prevention and Control maintains demographic data, and medical and reproductive histories were collected along with each blood sample. The goal of the serum bank is to provide specimens for prospective studies evaluating relations of serum concentrations of various analytes, such as hormones and antioxidant nutrients with breast cancer risk. Positive associations of bioavailable estradiol and testosterone with postmenopausal breast cancer have been found in these women.

Pittsburgh Cancer Institute Serum Bank and Tissue Bank

The Pittsburgh Cancer Institute (PCI) Serum and Tissue Bank is supported by the Department of Veterans Affairs and located at the VA Medical Center in Pittsburgh, Pennsylvania. The serum bank collects specimens and freezes sera for use in current and future studies. Surgically removed tumors are banked after informed consent is obtained. These specimens and accompanying data are available to PCI investigators and collaborating physicians in the community for clinical research.

Program for Critical Technologies in Breast Oncology

Yale University has established a core technical and tissue resource of human breast tissue. The goals of the tissue resource are to maximize access to human breast tissues and tumor DNA for researchers and to facilitate the application of molecular technologies in clinical breast cancer oncology. Breast tissue from patients treated at Yale New Haven Hospital and other hospitals in Connecticut is stored as fresh, fixed, or paraffin-embedded. A database has been established to support correlative multidisciplinary studies that utilize tissue samples.

Minimal fee-for-service routine molecular and histological tissue analyses of relevance to breast cancer are performed.

Program for Critical Technologies in Molecular Medicine

The Program for Critical Technologies in Molecular Medicine is a shared resource of the Yale Cancer Center, within the Department of Pathology at Yale University School of Medicine. The program was established in 1992, built on the existing tissue bank in the Department of Pathology. The Tissue Procurement Module and Tissue Products Module are two components of the program. The program is supported by several sources, including the G. Harold and Leila Y. Mathers Charitable Foundation, the NCI, the U.S. Army Medical Research and Materiel Command, and the Department of Pathology.

More than 10,000 frozen tissue samples have been collected for research purposes, and more than three million archived paraffin blocks from clinical cases are available. Tissue specimens are either frozen in OCT (optimum cutting temperature) or snap-frozen. Tissue specimens may also be formalin-fixed and paraffin-embedded for research use in addition to the paraffin blocks from archived clinical cases. Approximately 25,000 cases are archived from clinical paraffin blocks each year.

Each investigator interested in obtaining tissue from the program must have a protocol for tissue use approved by the Yale Human Investigation Committee. Investigators from outside of Yale must have a Material Transfer Agreement negotiated and signed before tissue can be released. Tissue products are provided as small sections, depending on the researcher's requests, rather than as bulk tissue, as a more efficient use of a valuable resources. Patient information disclosed with each tissue specimen includes age, sex, and pathology diagnosis. However, more information can be obtained after consultation with the investigator.

Prostate Cancer Tumor Bank

The Prostate Cancer Tumor Bank at the VA Medical Center in San Antonio, Texas, is funded by the Department of Veteran Affairs. The purpose of the Tumor Bank is to establish a high-quality bank of prostate tumors and an associated database of relevant clinical and follow-up data. The long-term goal for the banked tumor specimens is for use in studies for the discovery and validation of biological markers, such as oncoproteins and growth factors, which would correlate with clinical outcome and could be used as a prognostic indicator of tumor behavior.

Bank specimens are collected from excess tissue removed at biopsy or surgery. Fresh tumor specimens are snap-frozen in liquid nitrogen. In addition, archived paraffin-embedded material will be identified and assessed for potential use in immunohistochemical or molecular biological studies. The blocks are recut and reembedded if necessary and stored in the Tumor Bank under controlled conditions. Both abnormal and adjacent normal tissue is collected. More than 850 cases from paraffin-embedded archived tissues have been collected. Hematoxylin and eosin slides have been prepared, and tumor analysis has been performed and the data entered into the database. More than 180 specimens of fresh-frozen prostate tissue have been entered into the bank.

The database includes demographic, clinical, and outcome data for each specimen. Patient-specific data is obtained from existing sources, primarily hospital tumor registries, and thus, there is no direct patient contact. Access to banked material is strictly controlled, and use of specimens requires approval by the bank's executive committee.

Regional Tumor Bank

A regional tumor bank has been established at the VA Medical Center in Salt Lake City, Utah, and is supported by the Department of Veterans Affairs. Fresh tumor tissue will be snap-frozen and stored, and small samples will be stored as paraffin blocks. Tumor specimens will be available for future studies for current and future hypotheses regarding tumors.

Resource for Tumor Tissue and Data

The Resource for Tumor Tissue and Data at Kaplan Comprehensive Cancer Center, NYU School of Medicine, provides fresh human tissue specimens, data required for quality control as well as for correlation of research findings with clinical outcome, and identification of hospital patients with specific malignancies for administration of epidemiologic questionnaires and for recruitment for protocol studies. Services are provided free of charge. Tissue specimens can be either fixed or snap-frozen, according to the investigator's needs, and cell suspensions are also available. If no immediate need exists for tumor specimens obtained, these are stored and frozen until requested. Tissue paraffin blocks are available for immunophenotypic or immunogenotypic studies. Tumor and control blocks are provided to an investigator with a copy of the pathology report. Unused sections of the blocks must be returned on completion of the study.

Specialized Programs of Research Excellence

The Specialized Programs of Research Excellence (SPOREs) are highly inter-active, multidisciplinary programs of translational research directed at reducing the incidence, morbidity, and mortality of cancer. SPOREs are NCI-funded, NIH-Designated Clinical Research Centers at research universities and consist of cancer-specific research programs supported by core resources, including administration, tissue and serum banks, and biostatistics. SPOREs are designed to develop areas of basic science with potential impact on cancer and to move these promising areas into clinical trials. The SPOREs are also designed to communicate important findings rapidly into the research community to stimulate investigation and to bring validated translational findings into the medical community, where the research can ultimately reduce incidence and mortality of cancer. In 1993, NCI funded 22 SPOREs at a cost of almost $20 mil-lion—nine breast cancer, two gastrointestinal (colorectal and pancreatic can-cer), four lung cancer, and seven prostate cancer centers. Several SPOREs have core tissue banking facilities that support both their own research and collabo-ration with other SPOREs and researchers worldwide—for example, the SPORE in Prostate Cancer at the University of Michigan Comprehensive Cancer Center; SPOREs in Breast Cancer at Sloan-Kettering Institute for Cancer Research, Georgetown University Medical Center and Lombardi Cancer Center, and at Baylor College of Medicine in Houston; the SPORE in Lung Cancer at the University of Colorado Cancer Center; and SPOREs in Gastrointestinal Cancer and Prostate Cancer at Johns Hopkins.

Gastrointestinal. The SPORE in Gastrointestinal Cancer at Johns Hopkins is a translational research program aimed at reducing the incidence of and mortal-ity from colorectal and pancreatic cancer. The SPORE includes four research programs involving six projects supported by four core resources. All programs in this SPORE use human specimens. The Human Tissue Resource and Logis-tics Core, built on an existing bank established in 1986 for the Bowel Tumor Working Group, banks a wide range of tissues from resection specimens of colorectal and pancreatic cancers. By the end of 1995, the bank contained 910 colorectal cancer resections, 169 colorectal adenoma resections, 52 colorectal polypectomy specimens, 62 hepatic resections for metastatic colorectal cancer, 201 pancreatic cancer resections, 112 xenografts of pancreatic carcinoma, 127 fecal specimens, and 2,574 blood specimens. The core also provides for the procurement of fecal and blood specimens, including peripheral blood leuko-cytes, plasma and serum, nasogastric and duodenal capsule fluid, and peri-toneal washings. The core also maintains the Colorectal and Pancreatic Cancer Patient Registry. The registry is maintained in a database and includes family histories and food frequency questionnaires for patients evaluated for colo-rectal neoplasia. In addition, 2,120 families have been enrolled in the registry based on family history, including families with hereditary colorectal cancer syndromes and familial aggregation of colorectal cancer and early onset of colorectal cancer.

The University of Nebraska Medical Center Gastrointestinal Cancer SPORE largely focuses on issues in pancreatic cancer. There are no effective clinical approaches to prevention or early detection for pancreatic cancer. Therefore, this SPORE focuses on prevention, early detection, and therapy. The Nebraska SPORE consists of three cores designed to support existing research projects and provide for future research studies: Biostatistics, Tissue Bank, and the Pancreatic Cancer Family Registry. The tissue bank and family registry provide both normal and diseased pancreatic tissues for specialized studies and serve as a clinical resource for testing strategies for prevention and early detection approaches.

A Pancreas Tumor SPORE Tissue bank has been established to provide SPORE investigators with human specimens for translational research. The tissue bank will store normal, benign (acute and/or chronic fibrosing pancreatitis), and malignant pancreatic tissues (both primary and metastatic pancreatic carcinomas), peripheral blood lymphocytes, and plasma and serum from patients with pancreatic malignancies.

Prostate. The Prostate SPORE at Johns Hopkins takes a multidisciplinary approach to reduce the incidence, morbidity, and mortality of prostate cancer through prevention, genetics, early detection and diagnosis, morbidity reduction, and treatment. Research in early detection and diagnosis will be correlated with cancer risk in the Baltimore Longitudinal Study of Aging, the world's largest and longest longitudinal aging study (see Chapter Five). A large core tissue bank was established to accelerate translation of human prostate research to clinical medicine. The Prostate SPORE at Johns Hopkins is an interactive clinical and basic research team dedicated to translating new discoveries into the control of prostate cancer.

The goals of the University of Michigan Comprehensive Cancer Center (UMCCC) Prostate SPORE are to reduce the morbidity and mortality of prostate cancer by supporting and establishing a translational research program directed at understanding the biology of prostate cancer as well as developing new tools for the diagnosis, prevention, and treatment of prostate cancer. The UMCCC SPORE consists of multidisciplinary projects with emphasis on molecular and clinical epidemiology and novel therapeutics. Four cores support these research projects: administration, tissue and serum bank resource, animal and cell line models, and biostatistics. The Tissue and Serum Bank provides tissue and known clinical follow-up to evaluate chromosome alterations discovered in research studies in the SPORE.

The Prostate SPORE at Baylor College of Medicine provides researchers with resources to work toward the goal of reducing the incidence, morbidity, and mortality from prostate cancer. Five translational research objectives have been designed to expand successful intervention strategies against prostate cancer. Research projects include defining new markers of progression and metastasis, identifying novel methods for low-risk definitive therapy of early stage cancer, defining chemoprevention with such biologic agents as retinoids or vitamin D analogs, and designing treatment protocols for advanced disease with biologic agents.

Breast. The University of North Carolina (UNC) Lineberger Comprehensive Cancer Center SPORE in Breast Cancer currently consists of seven research projects and four core resources. The goal of the UNC SPORE is to reduce breast cancer mortality and incidence in North Carolina through an inter-disciplinary program of research. The UNC SPORE integrates studies in cancer prevention and control, molecular epidemiology, clinical research, and labora-tory clinical research. It also targets behavioral and biologic issues relevant to the African-American population. The tissue procurement and analysis core facility will provide tissue procurement, processing, and distribution services of breast tissue to SPORE investigators. The core accesses all breast surgical pro-cedures and obtains blood samples and fresh tissue. All collected tissues are entered into a database and may be distributed as DNA, RNA, or tissue sections to investigators.

The Carolina Breast Cancer Study, one of the seven research projects at the UNC SPORE, is a case-control study that integrates molecular biology and epi-demiology in the search for causes of breast cancer. Women from eastern and central North Carolina who are diagnosed with invasive breast cancer for the first time and who are between the ages of 20 and 74 are being recruited from September 1, 1995, to March 31, 2000. Comparison subjects will be frequency-matched by age and race. It is expected that 1,600 women with invasive breast cancer and an equal number of controls will be involved in the study. Blood samples will be collected for extraction of germ line DNA from all consenting participants, and paraffin-embedded tumor specimens will be requested for all breast cancer cases. Clinical data, stage, and prognostic characteristics will be collected with each specimen. This collection of specimens and data will be the basis for studies investigating the contributions of genes and the environment to breast carcinogenesis.

The SPORE in Breast Cancer at the Sloan-Kettering Institute for Cancer Research proposes to meet the needs of the oncologic community for an inte-grated clinical and laboratory setting committed to reducing the incidence of and mortality from breast cancer. The SPORE consists of five main research projects and two core resources. Research projects include studies of the erb family, BRCA-1, heregulin, and TGF-beta genes.

(Tissue banks at the Breast Cancer SPOREs at Georgetown University, Baylor College of Medicine, and Duke University are described in Table 3.1).

Lung. The goals of the University of Colorado Cancer Center (UCCC) Lung Cancer SPORE are to expand the understanding of the biology of lung cancer, to find new methods of diagnosis, prevention, and treatment, and to serve as a resource for the study of lung cancer. Since its inception, the UCCC SPORE has collected more than 900 sputum samples from high-risk individuals and more than 200 lung cancer specimens of all histologic types with matching pre- and postsurgical sputum samples for genetic testing of specific genes. During the next five years, the UCCC SPORE is planning to conduct eight interrelating full research projects, initiate four or five pilot projects annually, conduct more than 12 clinical trials, and support five core resources, including a premalignant and cancer bank. Specimens collected in the tissue banks will be available to scientists worldwide.

A Tissue Banks Core has been established to provide SPORE investigators well-preserved and well-characterized tumors, dysplastic lesions, benign tissues, cell lines, and cell and tissue fractions as well as associated clinical data for research projects. Tumor specimens, peripheral blood cells, urine, and sputum from patients with lung cancer or at risk for lung cancer will be collected. Tissue from invasive tumors and adjacent nonneoplastic lung tissue, pretreatment plasma, and peripheral blood cells from patients with these tumors are collected and processed from patients treated at SPORE-affiliated institutions. The Tissue Banks Core will thus serve as a national resource for uniformly typed, staged, treated, and observed tumors and preneoplastic lesions. Tissue specimens will be available to SPORE investigators and outside approved investigators.

Sloan-Kettering Institute

The Memorial Sloan-Kettering Cancer Center (MSKCC) was established in 1884 and is the oldest and largest private institution dedicated to the prevention, patient care, research, and education in cancer. MSKCC is composed of two institutes, Memorial Hospital and the Sloan-Kettering Institute. The Sloan-Kettering Institute is the basic science research facility and conducts innovative programs in biology, genetics, biochemistry, structural biology, immunology, and therapeutics. The Human Tissue Procurement and Tissue Bank Facility is one of the Core Research Facilities. It serves as a collection and distribution site for human tissue specimens to be used in MSKCC research projects.

The Soft Tissue Sarcoma (STS) Project within the Sloan-Kettering Institute is one of many ongoing research projects and is supported by the NCI. The STS project seeks to implement a comprehensive and integrated multidisciplinary program focused on the biology, pathogenesis, and natural history of soft tissue sarcoma and translate the research data into improved treatment strategies. The Pathology Core provides project investigators with fresh tissue surgical specimens and pathologic and histologic characterization of all soft tissue sarcoma cases from Memorial Hospital. The core also maintains a bank of frozen sarcoma tissue and provides tissue specimens for molecular, biochemical, and genetic studies. This tissue bank is one of the largest collections of its kind in the United States.

St. Louis University Alzheimer's Brain Bank

The Department of Geriatric Psychiatry at St. Louis University Health Sciences Center has established a community brain bank subsidized by the Alzheimer's Association. Almost 1,000 brains are stored at the brain bank. The brain bank specializes in degenerative brain diseases and dementias and is also involved in basic/clinical correlative research. Tissue samples are available to qualified investigators throughout the United States and abroad.

St. Paul- Ramsey Medical Center

A brain bank has been established at the St. Paul–Ramsey Medical Center in Minnesota. The brain bank currently contains frozen slices of brain tissue from more than 700 people with Alzheimer's disease and other forms of dementia. Tissue samples have been sent to Alzheimer's investigators at other institutions for research into the diagnosis, treatment, and cause of Alzheimer's disease.

Tissue Bank for Research on HIV-Associated Malignancies

A tissue bank for research on HIV-associated malignancies was established at the University Hospital of Downstate Medical Center in New York. The tissue bank is supported by the NCI. The goals of the tissue bank project are to maintain a central repository and database of neoplastic tissues and biological specimens of HIV-related malignancies with clinical and outcome data, to emphasize and prioritize the accrual of HIV-associated invasive and in-situ carcinoma of the uterine cervix, and to make available specimens for molecular, immunologic, genetic, and epidemiologic analysis to the scientific community. The participating institutions include the State University of New York Health Science Center at Brooklyn, King's County Hospital Center, and Woodhull Medical and Mental Health Center. Specimens may be shipped fresh to investigators, frozen as sterile, single-cell suspensions, or flash-frozen in a cryo-preservative reagent. Parallel paraffin blocks to frozen specimens are also made and stored.

Tissue Banking for Early Detection Research Network

The VA Medical Center in Pittsburgh, Pennsylvania, has established a tissue banking network that is supported by the Department of Veterans Affairs. Tissues from patients at risk for head, neck, and lung cancers will be obtained at surgery and stored in a tissue bank. These specimens will be used locally and distributed to requesting investigators at other institutions.

Tissue Core Facility at the Oral Cancer Research Center

The Oral Cancer Research Center of the University of Texas M.D. Anderson Cancer Center maintains a tissue core facility. The tissue core facility is supported by the National Institute of Dental Research. The core will function as a central repository for patient specimens, including peripheral blood lymphocytes for different projects in the Oral Cancer Research Center. The core is responsible for the acquisition, storage, and distribution of histologically characterized samples from various lesions representing the histopathological spectrum of oral squamous neoplasia.

Tissue Culture Core

The Tissue Culture Core at Weill Medical College of Cornell University serves as a common resource to provide specifically characterized cell cultures for faculty investigators. The Tissue Culture Core can provide human arterial smooth cell muscle cells, adventitial fibroblasts, umbilical vein endothelial cells, human monocyte-like cell lines, and peripheral blood monocytes. Fresh human platelets and neutrophils can be isolated per investigator request. All cell cultures are characterized immunocytochemically and tested for mycoplasma contamination.

Tissue/Pathology Core

The Tissue/Pathology Core is the central facility providing tissue collection and services for investigators of the University of Michigan Specialized Center of Research (SCOR). The core processes human lung tissue from patients with interstitial lung disease and controls for protein and mRNA analysis. Human bronchioalveolar lavage fluid and cells are also collected and processed for protein and mRNA analysis.

Tissue Procurement and Banking Facility

The Tissue Procurement and Banking Facility (TPBF) is an established CCSG-supported core facility at the University of Texas M.D. Anderson Cancer Center and is funded by the NCI. The TPBF provides human tumor tissues that have been removed for biopsy or therapeutic resections for ongoing research projects. The TPBF attempts to procure all pathologic tumor tissue from patient procedures for cryopreservation and characterizes tissues prior to distribution. Clinical data (epidemiology, family history, patient treatment, and patient outcome) for collected tissue specimens will be available through interactive databases.

Tissue Procurement Core

The Tissue Procurement Core at the University of Michigan Comprehensive Cancer Center (UMCCC) is funded by the NIC and the University of Michigan. The Tissue Procurement Core is a service of UMCCC based in the Surgical Pathology Laboratory of the University of Michigan Hospital. The Tissue Procurement Core prospectively obtains surgically resected tissue for research and maintains a –80°C freezer for limited storage. Tissue Procurement Core Services are available to UMCCC members only. For a nominal charge, histology services are available, including preparation of histologic sections from frozen and paraffin-embedded tissues, routine stains, and immunohistochemical stains. Acquisition of any tissue that is to be the subject of research or development requires IRB approval.

Tissue Procurement Core Facility

The Tissue Procurement Core Facility at Dartmouth College is designed to serve as a central tissue acquisition and distribution facility. Tissues are obtained from the reproductive tracts of patients undergoing hysterectomy or endometrial biopsy for program project investigators. Cell suspensions and vibratome sections are made from tissues of the fallopian tube, uterus, cervix, and vagina. Pertinent patient information from chart and patient interview and clinical/pathological evaluation of tissue specimens is collected.

Tissue Procurement Shared Resource

The Tissue Procurement Shared Resource (TPSR) at Ohio State University (OSU) Comprehensive Cancer Center was established as a shared service in 1975 to provide investigators with quality human tissue for research. TPSR obtains fresh tumor specimens to distribute around the world. The goals of the center are to provide an organized structure to access human tissue; to increase availability and diversity of tissues; to provide quality specimens, pathology data, and maintain patient confidentiality; and to maintain efficient and cost-effective service. The service has handled more than 75,000 specimens, approximately 3,000 per year. TPSR currently is funded by a Cancer Center Support Grant, OSU funds, and other grants. Investigators can receive remnant surgical or autopsy tissue after filling out a TPSR application. The application must have an approved human subjects IRB evaluation. All tissues are uniquely coded, and investigators receive a pathology report specifically about the tissue. For an additional fee, TPSR will perform a histology quality-control analysis on a small sample of the investigator's specimen.

Tumor Bank for Solid Tumors

The Tumor Bank for Solid Tumors at the Louisiana State University's Stanley S. Scott Cancer Center Tumor Bank, Department of Surgery, is supported by the Department of Veterans Affairs. All patients who have been previously scheduled for resection of malignancy are eligible to donate, and all tumor sites are collected. Aliquots of tumor and surrounding normal tissue are harvested. All tissue specimens are frozen, and routine pathology reports are collected with each specimen. Specimens are available for molecular analysis and correlative studies through the Stanley S. Scott Cancer Center. All tissue requests must have IRB approval and approval by the Director of the Louisiana State University Tumor Bank.

Western Genitourinary Tissue Bank

The Western Genitourinary Tissue Bank is located in the Department of Pathology at the University of Pittsburgh Medical Center (UPMC). The Tissue Bank was established in the early 1990s and has successfully banked over 250 prostatectomy specimens. The bank also stores serum and lymphocyte components for each individual collected prior to the radical prostatectomy surgery.

In addition to collecting specimens in house, a collaborative effort with the Veterans Affairs Medical Center in Pittsburgh also provides tissue specimens for the bank.

Wisconsin's Alzheimer's Disease Brain Tissue Bank

The Medical College of Wisconsin maintains an Alzheimer's Disease Brain Tissue Bank. More than 500 brain autopsies have been performed since its inception. Other tissue specimens and CSF samples from 267 cases are stored at –70°C. Brain and tissue specimens are from cases of Alzheimer's, Lewy body dementia, CJD, Huntington's, and normal controls. The brain bank no longer accepts brain tissue donations for research. All stored tissue specimens are available to investigators at the Medical College of Wisconsin and outside investigators on special request.

COMMERCIAL ENTERPRISES

Some commercial enterprises maintain tissue banks for proprietary use, while others establish banks for storage and distribution purposes. LifeSpan Bio-Sciences, Inc., is an example of a company that maintains a proprietary tissue bank and offers services using their tissue bank, while PathServe collects human tissues and organs to market them to the research community. Other commercial entities market products to facilitate analysis of human tissues—normal and diseased—such as Clontech. Materials with multiple tissue types, kits containing DNA/RNA samples, and even protein samples from human tissues are currently on the market. These types of products will most likely expand with the demand to find target disease genes and are useful to both academic and industry researchers.

LifeSpan BioSciences, Inc.

LifeSpan BioSciences, Inc., founded in 1995, is a genomics company focused on the discovery and licensing of genes that play a role in the aging process and identifying disease-associated genes for use as therapeutic or diagnostic targets. Because highly characterized samples of normal and diseased tissues are critical in localizing disease-associated genes, LifeSpan has an on-site tissue bank. LifeSpan's Tissue and Disease Bank contains one million normal and diseased human samples. The tissue bank has more than 175 different types of tissues from virtually every organ in the body, covering all ages. The tissue bank also includes more than 1,500 different pathologic disease categories, such as auto-immune diseases, infectious diseases, degenerative diseases, cancer and benign proliferative diseases, and genetic diseases. LifeSpan BioSciences, Inc., does not sell its tissues per se but performs custom services using its tissue bank.

LifeSpan BioSciences, Inc., performs a variety of services on its proprietary tissues, including high-throughput gene expression analysis, bioinformatics, immunocytochemistry and in situ hybridization (ICC/ISH), and anatomic mapping. ICC and ISH are customarily performed using one tissue per slide and are accompanied by a pathologic report of the lesion and the result from the test.

PathServe

PathServe Autopsy and Tissue Bank, established in 1990 and commercial since 1996, is a major supplier of human tissue to biotechnology and neuropathological research institutions. PathServe also serves as a main training facility of autopsy technicians for private pathologists and local hospitals. PathServe collects all types of organs and tissues, including placental and fetal specimens. Tissues are obtained through postmortem examinations, referrals from transplant banks of nontransplantable organs, and donations by next of kin. PathServe collects specimens from approximately 300 autopsies per year, and each autopsy yields approximately 100 specimens. PathServe has approximately 300 specimens stored at any one time and has distributed approximately 30,000 specimens in the last year. Consent for donation is obtained from the family. PathServe does not maintain a centralized storage facility. Instead, specimens are stored in the morgues of different hospitals.

Clontech

Clontech was established in 1984 as a developer and marketer of biological products to the life sciences market worldwide. Clontech's mission is to accelerate the discovery process by providing innovative tools that enable researchers to answer complex questions more expediently. Clontech was the first to make several key technologies available to the biomedical field, including the green fluorescence protein-based reporter system, two-hybrid analysis systems for the study of protein interactions, and gene array technology for high-throughput differential expression analysis. Such recent products as RNA Master Blots and high-quality protein samples facilitate screening of normal and diseased human tissues from multiple organs. These products enable researchers to profile tissue expression patterns of known genes or expressed sequence tags (ESTs), to obtain high-throughput analysis of gene expression profiles in different tissues, and to perform rapid screenings of tissue-specific patterns of genes.

NONPROFIT ORGANIZATIONS (NONEDUCATIONAL)

A variety of nonprofit institutions bank tissues for storage and distribution. Nonprofit institutions, such as the American Type Culture Collection, Coriell Institute for Medical Research, the Research Foundation for Mental Hygiene, the Rocky Mountain Multiple Sclerosis Center, the National Psoriasis Tissue Bank, the Kaiser Permanente Center for Health Research, and the Hereditary Disease Foundation, receive millions of dollars in federal funding. Descriptions of these nonprofit centers that bank tissue are detailed below.

American Type Culture Collection

Since its establishment in 1925, the American Type Culture Collection (ATCC) has served as an archive of living cultures and genetic materials for researchers in the biological sciences. The mission of the ATCC is to acquire, authenticate, and maintain reference cultures, related biological materials, and associated data and to distribute these to qualified scientists in government, industry, and education. The ATCC has approximately 2,300 human cell lines. All of the human cell lines are immortalized cultures and the genetic material is mainly the products of recombinant DNA research. ATCC is creating new products to facilitate screening of multiple cell lines/tissue types. For example, the ATCC Express-Check is a kit that contains DNA from human tissue-specific cDNA libraries.

Biologic Specimen Bank

The Research Institute on Addictions in New York has established a biologic specimen bank to support scientific research projects at the institute. The bank will collect and store frozen specimens of plasma, serum, cells, cell membranes, and urine from randomly selected African-American and Caucasian men and women, aged 35 to 79. Control tissue specimens will be collected from two case-control studies on myocardial infarction and lung cancer and participants in the research component project on the epidemiology of treated and untreated alcoholics. Blood samples from more than 7,500 men and women are expected to be collected and stored.

Biomedical Research Institute

The Biomedical Research Institute is a nonprofit entity established in 1948 to provide research and development services. The Biomedical Research Institute specializes in tropical disease vaccines and provides biological repository services to federal agencies. The National Institute of Child Health and Human Development (NICHD) is conducting a trial of calcium supplementation in pregnancy. The Biomedical Research Institute will store, monitor, and distribute serum, plasma, and urine samples collected from this trial. More than 4,500 pregnant women are expected to enroll in this study from five clinical centers. NICHD has also contracted with the Biomedical Research Institute for banking blood specimens in a similar fashion for two other studies: Diabetes in Early Pregnancy and Successive Small-for-Gestational-Age Birth.

Coriell Institute for Medical Research

The Coriell Institute for Medical Research is a basic biomedical research institution that conducts research on the causes of genetic diseases, including cancer. The Coriell Institute's three missions are research, cell banking, and public education. The largest collection of human cells for research is maintained at the Coriell Institute, and these cells are available to the general scientific community. Seminal research on the genes associated with Huntington's disease, cystic fibrosis, Alzheimer's disease, ataxia telangiectasia, and manic depression have utilized cells from the Coriell collection. In 1990, the NIMH awarded the Coriell Institute a $5.7 million contract to establish a cell repository for the study of the genetic basis of Alzheimer's disease, manic depression and schizophrenia. New repositories have recently been established for the study of diabetes.

The Coriell Cell Repositories are supported by NIH and several foundations. More than 35,000 cell lines are currently stored, representing approximately 1,000 of the 4,000 known genetic diseases, and 60,000 cell lines have been distributed to more than 40 nations, resulting in 8,000-plus research publications. Cultures are established from both blood and skin, and the cells are stored frozen at the institute. Three-quarters of a million vials of cells are kept in 37 giant liquid nitrogen tanks. The Coriell Cell Repositories currently consist of four cell collections described below.

Human Genetic Mutant Cell Repository. The Human Genetic Mutant Cell Repository is sponsored by the National Institute of General Medical Sciences (NIGMS). The repository supplies scientists with materials for advancing the discovery of disease-related genes. Their resources include highly characterized, viable, contaminant-free cell cultures and high-quality DNA derived from these cultures. The repository contains both DNA and cell cultures from human and animal cell cultures, normal controls, inherited disorders and normal variants, and NIGMS extended family collections.

NIA Aging Cell Repository. The NIA Aging Cell Repository is a collection set up to facilitate cellular and molecular research studies on the mechanisms of aging and degenerative processes. Included in the collection are cell cultures from aging syndromes, Alzheimer's, normal fibroblasts from a lifetime study, lymphoblasts for aged sib pairs, and a variety of other cell types.

American Diabetes Association (ADA) Cell Repository Maturity Onset Diabetes Collection. The ADA Cell Repository Maturity Onset Diabetes Collection is derived from the ADA Genetics of non–insulin dependent diabetes mellitus/NIDDM (GENNID) Study. The purpose of the study is to establish a national database and cell repository consisting of information and genetic material from families with well-documented NIDDM. The repository contains DNA samples and phenotypic data from subjects enrolled in Phase I ADA GENNID trials (170 pedigrees, all of which contain at least one affected sib pair, with a total of 650 affected individuals and approximately 1,200 subjects). The data set includes multiple metabolic factors, such as carbohydrate metabolism, lipid metabolism, and body size measures, as well as lifestyle variables. New additions to the collection include families and pedigrees, sib pairs, and DNA samples from Phase II of the ADA GENNID study.

Human Biological Data Interchange Cell Repository Juvenile Diabetes Collection. The Human Biological Data Interchange (HBDI) Cell Repository Juvenile Diabetes Collection contains quality-controlled cell lines and DNA from more than 400 families for distribution.

Fox Chase Network Breast Cancer Risk Registry

The Fox Chase Network Breast Cancer Risk Registry is supported by the Department of the Army. The goal of the registry is to establish a breast cancer risk registry to serve as a resource for research activities investigating the etiology and prevention of breast cancer. Women with one or more first-degree relatives with breast cancer are identified, and information about family history, personal medical history, lifestyle and environmental factors, health practices and beliefs, and psychological status are entered into a comprehensive database. Serum and DNA from women in this high-risk registry are stored in the Fox Chase Cancer Center/Network Breast Cancer Tissue Registry. In addition, a high-risk specimen bank contains DNA, red blood cells, plasma, and breast tissue.

HealthPartners Human Brain Bank

The HealthPartners Human Brain Bank in Minnesota was established by Dr. William Frey in 1977. The brain bank is supported by the Regions Hospital Foundation, pharmaceutical companies, and other private foundations and individuals. The brain bank contains frozen human brains from cases of Alzheimer's disease, multi-infarction dementia, dementia with Lewy bodies, Parkinson's disease, Pick's disease, CJD, unclassified dementias, and non-demented normal controls. More than 2,000 brain specimens have been collected. These brain specimens are available to collaborating investigators.

Hereditary Disease Foundation

The Hereditary Disease Foundation of Santa Monica, California, is studying the genes involved in Huntington's disease in a Venezuelan kindred of more than

14,000 people. Through study of this kindred, the gene for Huntington's disease was localized to chromosome 4p. This kindred is a valuable resource, enabling researchers to study members who share background genes and a common environment. The Hereditary Disease Foundation is studying the unstable trinucleotide (CAG) repeat found in the Huntington's disease gene. Huntington's disease has afflicted more than 400 people and now threatens 4,697 at-risk children in this kindred. To study this protein, the Hereditary Disease Foundation is collecting tissue samples, including lymphoblast lines and sperm samples, to examine the effect of age, disease duration, birth order, and environmental factors on sperm. Brain and other postmortem tissues from genetically and clinically well-characterized members of the kindred are also being collected to understand how the Huntington protein specifically devastates striatal neurons.

The International Skeletal Dysplasia Registry

The International Skeletal Dysplasia Registry at Cedars-Sinai Medical Center in California is a referral center for the diagnosis and management of skeletal dysplasias. The registry is supported by grants from NIH and the Steven Spielberg Pediatric Research Center. Materials submitted to the registry are archived and used for future research studies. Samples collected include histology blocks and slides, frozen and fixed tissue specimens, cell cultures (including fibroblasts, chondrocytes, and lymphoblastoid cells), blood (from patient and both parents), and DNA. Clinical summaries, pedigrees, photographs, and x-rays are also collected.

Kaiser Permanente Center for Health Research

The Kaiser Permanente Center for Health Research (CHR) is a nonprofit healthcare research institute established in 1964. More than 40 studies are under way and some involve the storage of tissue. For example, the CHR started the Benign Breast Disease Registry (BBDR), funded by the NCI. The BBDR includes data on nearly 10,000 women diagnosed between 1970 and 1994. The registry provides both benign and malignant archived tissue to researchers. In another NCI-sponsored breast cancer study, almost 16,000 breast cancer cases and associated archived tissue are available to qualified researchers for molecular studies. In the last 20 years, more than 25,000 people in the Portland-Vancouver area have voluntarily participated in the research at the CHR. Clinical trials involving archived tissue are also undertaken. For instance, the Fracture Intervention Trial is an 11-center double-blind, placebo-controlled, randomized clinical trial to determine the efficacy of alendronate in preventing fractures secondary to osteoporosis. The CHR has received more than $96 million in grants from federal and state agencies and private foundations.

Maryland Brain Collection

The Maryland Brain Collection (MBC) is a collaboration between the Maryland Psychiatric Research Center and the Office of the Chief Medical Examiner of Maryland. The MBC collects material for investigators interested in studying the aspects of human postmortem brain structure and function. Specimens are collected from deceased persons with schizophrenia, suicide victims, and healthy controls. Extensive clinical information is also obtained with each specimen and is available to investigators.

McKesson BioServices

McKesson BioServices, formerly Ogden BioServices Corporation, was established in 1986 to provide a cost-effective and focused process in several areas of drug development, such as regulatory affairs, formulation development, and biological specimen storage and distribution. McKesson BioServices currently stores more than 20 million biological specimens in their Biological Specimens Repository. Some of the nationally known collections of biological specimens stored by McKesson BioServices are briefly described in Table 3.2.

National Disease Research Interchange

The National Disease Research Interchange (NDRI) is a nonprofit organization that arranges for the procurement and distribution of human tissues and organs for biomedical researchers. NDRI has been operating for 17 years and has provided more than 125,000 tissue specimens of more than 100 types of tissues to scientists nationwide. NDRI is composed of three programs with different objectives to facilitate the use of human tissues and organs for researchers:

- Human Tissues and Organs for Research (HTOR): This unit focuses on retrieval and distribution of tissues and organs from autopsy and surgical procedures, as well as specimens obtained from eye and tissue banks. Examples include whole or partial organs, such as heart, lung, kidney, brain, liver, eyes, and bones and joints.

- Human Biological Data Interchange (HBDI): This unit stores genetically valuable family collections for use in the advancement and study of the genetic basis for disease. The HBDI repository currently holds biomaterials from more than 500 families and also contains family and medical history data on more than 6,500 families with diabetes.

- Odyssey One: This unit was established to respond to new and emerging needs of biomedical researchers in innovative areas related to the use of human materials in research. The unique and hard-to-get tissues that they have provided include pancreatic islet cells, malignant tumors and normal adjacent tissue, and bone marrow stem cells.

Table 3.2

McKesson BioServices- Biological Specimen Repository

Collection	Description
Army-Navy Serum Repository (ANSR)	The ANSR contains more than 18 million sera specimens collected from active-duty and reserve personnel. This repository is the largest collection of normal human sera from all race and ethnic groups and all geographic areas in the United States. This repository provides the Army with a seroepidemiology resource to assess exposure to infectious and toxic agents during deployment, to estimate immunity prevalence for a variety of diseases, and to determine the causes of, risk factors for, and determinants of acute and chronic diseases associated with military operations.
NHLBI-sponsored studies	The National Heart, Lung, and Blood Institute (NHLBI) contracts with McKesson BioServices to maintain a repository of blood specimens from NHLBI-sponsored studies. These specimens will be made available to investigators for research projects related to transfusion-transmitted diseases and a variety of other disorders of blood or the cardiovascular system. A serum, plasma, and cell repository is maintained and serologic and virologic assays are performed.
Collaborative Perinatal Project (CPP) Serum Repository	The CPP was a prospective cohort study of pregnancy and child development administered by the National Institute of Neurological and Communicative Disorders (NINCD). The purpose of the project was to enroll pregnant women between 1959 and 1966 and conduct follow-up neurological, psychological, pediatric, and speech-hearing studies on the children to determine factors responsible for the development of neurological disorders of childhood. The CPP collected serum from the women during pregnancy, delivery, and postpartum, and umbilical cord serum from the newborns, and serum from the infant at 4 months of age. More than 833,000 vials of serum were collected.
Diet Intervention Study in Children (DISC) Study Effort	The objectives of the DISC project are to determine whether a fat-modified diet during childhood and adolescence will lower LDL-cholesterol and to assess the feasibility and safety of this diet. The DISC project is being conducted at 6 clinical centers and a coordinating center. More than 600 children, between the ages of 8 and 10 who had LDL-cholesterol levels between the 80th and 98th percentiles and other criteria were randomized into the intervention or control group. Serum samples were collected at baseline and 12, 36, 37, 60, and 84 months and at 18 years of age after follow-up.

Table 3.2- **continued**

Collection	Description
National Health and Nutrition Examination Survey (NHANES) Serum Bank	The CDC NHANES project is a national probability sample survey program serving as a source of data obtained by standardized health examinations. Serum has been drawn from over 30,000 participants and stored at –80°C for future studies. These samples are available to government agencies and for other approved sociodemographic studies.
Polyp Prevention Trial (PPT)	The PPT is a multicentered randomized clinical study to determine if a low-fat, high-fiber, vegetable-, and fruit-enriched diet would decrease the rate of recurrence of large bowel adenomatous polyps. Under subcontract with Westat, Inc., McKesson BioServices provides biological repository services involving blood and tissue/biopsy specimen receipt, cataloging, storage, and inventory control.
Vaccine Evaluations	The NICHD conducts the Group B Streptococcus Study. McKesson BioServices is subcontracted by Westat, Inc., to provide biological repository services. An estimated 65,000 vials of serum and isolates will be collected and stored by McKesson BioServices sent by participating clinical centers. A computerized inventory system will be established for tracking and retrieval of all specimens.

National Neurological Research Specimen Bank

The National Neurological Research Specimen Bank (NNRSB) was established in 1961 to provide a vital resource to neuroscientists. The NNRSB is supported by NINDS/NIMH, the Department of Veterans Affairs, and private organizations, such as the National Multiple Sclerosis Society. The NNRSB at the VA Medical Center in Los Angeles, California, collects, cryogenically stores, and distributes donated tissue to research scientists around the world. The specimen bank stores pre- and postmortem tissues and cerebrospinal fluid/blood and other neurological specimens from patients with multiple sclerosis, Huntington's disease, Parkinson's disease, Alzheimer's disease, and HIV/AIDS.

National Psoriasis Tissue Bank

The National Psoriasis Tissue Bank (NPTB) is the only international public source of genetic material for psoriasis research. The bank is dedicated to finding the genetic causes of psoriasis and psoriatic arthritis. The stored tissue is available for use by international experts. The NPTB is supported by private donations through the National Psoriasis Foundation (NPF), a voluntary nonprofit national health agency. The NPTB consists of nearly 300 Epstein-Barr virus (EBV)–transformed cell lines, isolated DNA, fibroblasts from families with psoriasis and psoriatic arthritis, and blood samples from sibling pairs providing an additional 1,000 DNA samples. Researchers can obtain the cell line, DNA, family history, and medical history of any individual in the bank; however, names and locations of contributors remain anonymous. There is a small fee for the service. Blood and skin samples are obtained by a medical team at the Baylor Psoriasis Center, a regional referral Center at Baylor University Medical Center in Dallas, Texas.

New York State Multiple Sclerosis Consortium

The New York State Multiple Sclerosis Consortium brings together research and clinical expertise of 15 major medical centers in New York in an effort to further define the multiple sclerosis (MS) population in terms of demographic, clinical, functional, quality-of-life, and treatment parameters. The Department of Neurology at Buffalo General Hospital is the coordinating center for the New York State MS Consortium. Current research efforts involve the development of an MS patient registry and centralized database of MS patient information and the collection of specimens, including blood, tissue, and cerebrospinal fluid, for member centers. Tissue specimens are stored at the Baird Multiple Sclerosis and Neuroimmunology Tissue Repository, which was established in 1991 and is funded by a grant from the Baird Foundation to the Millard Fillmore Health, Education, and Research Foundation. The repository has collected more than 1,000 tissues and fluids from MS patients, along with detailed demographic and neurologic data.

Rocky Mountain Multiple Sclerosis Center Tissue Bank

The Rocky Mountain Multiple Sclerosis Center (RMMSC) Tissue Bank, one of the largest MS tissue banks in the world, was established in 1976 to procure, process, preserve, and distribute MS brain tissue to research laboratories from all over the world involved in finding the cause of and cure for MS. More than 170 CNS samples have been banked at RMMSC, representing material from a well-defined patient population. The stored tissue has led to several key discoveries in the pathogenesis of MS. The bank is funded by the National Multiple Sclerosis Society.

St. Luke's- Roosevelt Institute for Health Sciences

The Neuropathology Core at St. Luke's–Roosevelt Institute for Health Sciences has established a bank of CNS tissues from children who died with HIV-1 infection. The tissue bank is supported by the NINDS. Snap-frozen tissue blocks have been collected from 25 cases, and formalin-fixed, paraffin-embedded tissue blocks have been stored from these cases and from an additional 50 cases. Tissues will also be collected from HIV-1 negative control cases and HIV-1–

infected and negative adults. Tissue specimens are available to core investigators from the Neuropathology Division of Columbia-Presbyterian Medical Center. The core provides neuropathology support and tissue immunocytochemistry services.

The Stanley Brain Collection and Neuropathology Consortium

The Stanley Brain Collection and Neuropathology Consortium was set up in 1994 and is privately funded by the Theodore and Vada Stanley Foundation. Its mission is to make postmortem brain tissue from individuals with schizophrenia, bipolar disorder, major depression, and normal controls available for scientific investigations. The Stanley Foundation supports approximately half of all research in the United States directly related to bipolar disorder. The Stanley Foundation Brain Collection obtains brains through designated medical examiners in several cities. The brains are then forwarded to the NIMH Neuroscience Center at St. Elizabeth's Hospital in Washington, D.C. More than 200 brains have been collected so far and hospital and outpatient records are obtained with each brain to establish a firm diagnosis. All brains are fixed in a uniform matter: Half of the brain is frozen, and the other half is formalin-fixed. Selected areas of the brain thought to be involved in severe psychiatric disorders (e.g., hippocampus, basal ganglia, and prefrontal cortex) are dissected out and then sectioned into thin slices that are fixed to a glass slide.

The Stanley Foundation Neuropathology Consortium is a collection of 60 brains. The collection consists of four sets of 15 brains each from persons with schizophrenia, bipolar disorder, depression, and normal controls. The four sets are matched for age (mean age is 40), sex, race, side of brain, postmortem interval, and quality of brain DNA.

There are four main goals of the Stanley Foundation Neuropathology Consortium. The first is to make brain tissue from individuals with severe psychiatric disorders available to researchers. Secondly, different laboratories can measure the same thing in this uniform brain collection and be able to compare results. Thirdly, the consortium attempts to provide a composite picture of what is wrong in the brains of these individuals and how each differs from normal controls. Lastly, the consortium will be able to compare results on the brains of individuals with schizophrenia, bipolar disorder, severe depression, and normal controls to determine differences and similarities.

The 60 consortium brains are available at no charge to researchers worldwide. The brain specimens are distributed coded so that the research is conducted as a blind study. When the research is completed, the results are sent to Washington, and the codes are then sent to the investigators.

State of Florida Brain Bank

A brain bank was established by the State of Florida in 1985 and is supported by state funds. The bank was established as part of the state's Alzheimer's Disease Initiative (ADI), which supports research, service, and training in Alzheimer's disease and related memory disorders. The objectives of the ADI Brain Bank are to provide tissue for Alzheimer's disease research, to establish a diagnosis for use in clinical and pathological studies, and to provide families with a confirmed diagnosis. The bank is at the Mount Sinai Medical Center in Miami, Florida, and thirteen institutes in the state serve as sources of brains.

Brain tissue specimens are stored either frozen or fixed and more than 1,000 brains have been autopsied and stored. Tissue specimens are available to approved investigators at no cost.

Tissue Accrual and In Situ Imaging Core

The Wistar Institute maintains a tissue accrual and in situ imaging core to collect tissue specimens from melanomas, nevi, and blood samples. The core is supported by the NCI. The core has one of the largest collections of primary melanocytic cell cultures and freshly isolated DNA collections from these tissues. The core also has access to human tissue biopsies, including thousands of pigmented lesions from affiliated laboratories, such as Surgical Pathology (20,000 accessions per year).

Tumor Bank Facility at the Herbert Irving Comprehensive Cancer Center

The Tumor Bank Facility at Columbia-Presbyterian Medical Center's Herbert Irving Comprehensive Cancer Center in New York was established in 1972 to maximize investigational use of human tissues removed at surgery or autopsy. The core facility provides a mechanism for optimal collection, examination, and distribution of all human tissues for investigative purposes. The Tumor Bank contains both "targeted" and "nontargeted" specimens. The nontargeted specimens are tumors and tumor/normal tissue pairs collected and cryopreserved in substantial numbers. Most tissue specimens are snap-frozen to facilitate subsequent preparation of frozen sections for histology, immunohistochemistry, and other types of analyses and to preserve tissue for DNA/RNA isolation. Columbia-Presbyterian Cancer Center members may request specific tissues types. Users of the Tumor Bank Facility must be members of the Herbert Irving Comprehensive Cancer Center, and there is no charge for the specimens.

Chapter Four

TUMOR REGISTRIES

A tumor registry is a cancer data system that provides continued follow-up care on all cancer patients in a given location, hospital, or state. A tumor registry documents and stores all significant elements of a patient's history and treatment. Many registry databases include information concerning demographics, medical history, diagnostic findings, primary site, histological type of cancer, stage of disease, treatment(s), recurrence, subsequent treatment, and end results. A variety of studies and reports can be generated from the information contained in tumor registries.

Several registries also collect patient specimens, such as blood samples or slides of resected tumors. These specimens may be used for educational purposes as case studies or for research purposes. Several tumor registries that collect tissue specimens are described below as well as some of the larger tumor registries. For a more complete listing of tumor registries, see Appendix F.

THE NATIONAL FAMILIAL PANCREAS TUMOR REGISTRY

The National Familial Pancreas Tumor Registry was established in 1994 at Johns Hopkins Hospital in Maryland. The goals of the registry include documenting whether or not neoplasms of the pancreas occur in families, evaluating selected families to gain a better understanding of the genetic basis for development of carcinoma of the pancreas, and serving as a resource to other investigators interested in pancreatic cancer. Currently, 131 families have been entered into the registry. Families referred to the registry will be asked to fill out a questionnaire, and medical records and pathology slides of each affected family member are reviewed to confirm all cases. Blood samples are drawn from selected cases for genetic analysis. The registry is currently supported by private donors.

CALIFORNIA TUMOR TISSUE REGISTRY

The California Tumor Tissue Registry is a nonprofit organization committed to the enhancement of patient care. It was established in 1947 and was first funded by the California Medical Association. The registry is at the Loma Linda University School of Medicine in California. The goals of the registry are to educate and improve patient care, to provide high-quality consultation, and to serve as a resource for rare tumors. Through its education program, the registry provides subscribers with slides of rare and unusual tumors. A repository is maintained by the registry with more than 30,000 accessions and 30,000 consultations. Although the registry's influence is predominantly in California, it has provided materials to several other states, countries, and pathology teaching programs.

NCI COOPERATIVE FAMILY REGISTRY FOR BREAST CANCER STUDIES AND NCI COOPERATIVE FAMILY REGISTRY FOR COLORECTAL CANCER STUDIES

The Cooperative Family Registry for Breast Cancer Studies (CFRBCS), initiated by the NCI in 1995, contains biological specimens from patients with a family history of breast cancer, breast/ovarian cancer, or Li-Fraumeni syndrome and from their relatives. Six CFRBCS sites collaborate to ascertain families at high and intermediate risk for breast cancer.[1] Specimens are in the form of tissue sections from paraffin-embedded breast and ovarian cancers, peripheral blood lymphocytes, serum, fresh-frozen tissue, and other biological fluids. The CFRBCS provides related family history (pedigrees), clinical, demographic, and epidemiologic data on risk factors exposures but will not provide patient identification. In addition, the CFRBCS provides follow-up epidemiologic data as well as data on recurrence, new morbidity, and mortality from participating families. The CFRBCS repository and related databases are available to researchers to provide a resource for interdisciplinary and translational breast cancer research.

The Cooperative Family Registry for Colorectal Cancer Studies, a similar resource for colorectal cancer, was established in 1998. NCI supports six registries throughout the world including four in the United States: the University of Washington in Seattle, the University of Hawaii, the Mayo Clinic in Min-

---

[1]The six CFRBCS collaborating sites are the Australian Breast Cancer Family Registry, the Metropolitan New York Registry of Breast Cancer Families, the Northern California Cooperative Family Registry, the Ontario Registry for Studies of Familial Breast Cancer, the Philadelphia Familial Breast Cancer Registry, and the Utah Cooperative Breast Cancer Registry.

nesota, and the University of Southern California. These registries perform several tasks, including assembling and maintaining comprehensive lists of families with histories of colon cancer, collecting detailed information about possible factors involved in the cancer process, and serving as a storehouse of blood samples and tumor biopsies from family members for research purposes. The data and samples collected at any of these registries are available to investigators worldwide.

FAMILIAL BRAIN TUMOR REGISTRY

The mission of the Familial Brain Tumor Registry is to identify families who are at high risk for brain tumors and multiple cancer. The Familial Brain Tumor Registry is located at the University of Texas M.D. Anderson Cancer Center. The registry serves as a resource of families at high risk of cancer and allows for the study of genetic factors associated with the disease. Enrollment of families requires the occurrence of a brain tumor and another cancer in the immediate family. A short interview is conducted with the family to obtain a detailed family history of cancer. Blood samples or buccal smears are collected from family members.

SURVEILLANCE, EPIDEMIOLOGY, AND END RESULTS PROGRAM

The Surveillance, Epidemiology, and End Results (SEER) Program was established in 1971 and is supported by NCI. The goals of the SEER Program include assembling and reporting estimates of cancer incidence and mortality in the United States; monitoring annual cancer incidence trends to identify unusual changes in specific forms of cancer occurring in population subgroups; providing continuing information on changes over time in disease, trends in therapy, and patient survival rates; and promoting studies designed to identify factors amenable to cancer-control interventions, such as dietary or environmental exposures, screening practices, and treatment practices.

The SEER Program collects cancer data on a routine basis from designated population-based cancer registries in nine areas of the United States. The geographic areas represent an estimated 14 percent of the U.S. population. Trends in cancer incidence, mortality, and patient survival as well as many other studies are derived from the SEER database. The database contains information on approximately 2.3 million in situ and invasive cancers diagnosed between 1973 and 1996, with approximately 125,000 new cases accessioned each year.

NEW YORK STATE CANCER REGISTRY

The New York State Cancer Registry in Albany, New York, is administered by the New York State Department of Health with supporting funds from the Centers for Disease Control and Prevention. The registry collects, processes, and reports information about every New Yorker diagnosed with cancer. The New York State Cancer Registry is one of the oldest cancer registries in the country and has been collecting information on patients with cancer for more than 50 years.

The Cancer Registry includes reports of all malignant cancers, except selected skin cancers. The Cancer Registry receives more than 135,000 case reports each year, representing more than 83,000 new tumors. It collects data on the anatomic site of the tumor, the stage of diagnosis, morphology, and treatment information. It also collects specific sociodemographic information on each individual. In total, more than 100 different pieces of information on each person are collected.

Chapter Five

TISSUE COLLECTIONS CREATED FROM LONGITUDINAL AND INDIVIDUAL RESEARCH STUDIES

Research on human disease or human physiology has long required the examination of human tissue from multiple research subjects. Tissues from both affected patients and normal controls are necessary for comparison studies to ascertain the etiology and pathology of a particular disease. By studying diseased tissue, researchers can delineate the normal pathway and understand the mechanisms underlying growth, development, and function. Thus, an advantage exists in obtaining tissue from affected persons for scientific study.

In a world where time and money are scarce, it is extremely costly for researchers who require tissue samples from a select group to wait for these persons to enter their hospitals or clinics. Often, different research projects may require the same set of tissue samples. This chapter briefly describes several research studies that have already collected or are continuing to collect human tissue samples. Depending on how these tissues were obtained, they may be available for other research studies.

LONGITUDINAL STUDIES

Longitudinal studies, in which the same group of individuals is studied at intervals over a prolonged period, often collect large numbers of specimens that can be used for both retrospective and prospective research. Several well-known longitudinal studies have been conducted over the years, including the Physicians' Health Study, the Nurses' Health Study, and the Framingham Heart Study. Other large longitudinal studies include the Women's Health Initiative, the Health Professionals Follow-Up Study, the MRFIT study, and the National Health and Nutrition Examination Surveys. Several longitudinal studies are described below.

The National Institutes of Health Women's Health Initiative

The NIH Women's Health Initiative (WHI), established in 1991, is the largest preventive study of women's health in the United States. The WHI is a 15-year research program, concluding in 2005, that focuses on the major causes of death, disability, and impaired quality of life in postmenopausal women. The overall goal of WHI is to reduce coronary heart disease, breast and colorectal cancer, and osteoporosis in postmenopausal women through prevention, intervention, and risk factor identification.

The WHI will involve more than 168,000 women of all races and socioeconomic backgrounds aged 50–79. Recruitment began in September 1993 and concluded in January 1998. The WHI conducts three studies: a randomized clinical trial, an observation study, and a community prevention study. Almost 70,000 women are enrolled in the randomized clinical trial that consists of three study groups: hormone replacement therapy, dietary modification, and calcium and vitamin D supplementation. Eligible women could choose to be in one, two, or all three of the study groups. The observational study will track the medical history and health habits of approximately 100,000 women to examine the relationship between lifestyle, health and risk factors, and disease. The clinical trial and observational study are conducted at 40 clinical centers nationwide. The Fred Hutchinson Cancer Research Center in Seattle, Washington, is the WHI Clinical Coordinating Center for data collection, management, and analysis.

The 168,000 women enrolled in both the clinical trial and the observational study will be followed for eight to 12 years and will provide multiple blood samples throughout the course of the study. Participants sign a consent form that states that the collection of blood samples is for use in future research, which may include genetic research, and participants will not be informed of any test results. Participants may opt out of having their samples used for genetic research if they so desire. The clinical trial participants provide a blood sample at their initial visit and at their one-year visit, and a subset of participants have samples drawn at three, six, and nine years. Blood samples are also collected from participants in the observational trial at their initial visit, and then again at their three-year visit. Blood samples are divided into serum, plasma, and buffy coat and are stored at a central facility in Rockville, Maryland. Participants' charts contain identifying information, including name, Social Security number, and address and telephone number, which are barcoded. Blood samples are labeled with matching bar codes to link them to the charts. Approximately 27,000 women will be enrolled in the hormone replacement therapy trial, some of whom will also undergo an endometrial biopsy to rule out endometrial hyperplasia or cancer.[1] These biopsies are stored at the individual clinical centers within the pathology departments and are labeled with a pathology accession number. In cases where abnormalities are detected, slides of the biopsy are bar-coded and sent to a central laboratory at NIH. Participants and their physicians are informed of any abnormalities found in the endometrial biopsy. All study records will be kept indefinitely for analysis and follow-up.

The third component of the WHI, the community prevention study, is a five-year collaborative effort with the Centers for Disease Control and Prevention (CDC) to study community approaches to developing healthy behaviors. This study will include women of all races and socioeconomic backgrounds, aged 40 and over. Eight university-based prevention centers will conduct and evaluate health programs that encourage women to adopt improved diet, nutritional supplementation, smoking cessation, exercise, and early detection of treatable health problems, among other healthy behaviors.

Baltimore Longitudinal Study of Aging

The Longitudinal Studies Branch of the NIA is responsible for the operation and management of the Baltimore Longitudinal Study of Aging. The Baltimore Longitudinal Study was initiated in 1958, enrolling only men until 1978, when women were included. The Longitudinal Studies Branch has a research program based primarily on the Baltimore Longitudinal Study because it offers a unique opportunity to study a number of aging-related diseases and disabilities, including frailty, Alzheimer's disease, cardiovascular disease, cancer, osteoporosis, and menopause.

Storage of blood samples and blood fractions began in 1963 and has been systematically continued since. Serum, plasma, lyophilized erythrocytes and whole-blood plasma (including leukocytes), and aliquots of 24-hour urine collections have all been stored. Over the years, samples have been used for various approved protocols. For example, a longitudinal study of prostate-specific antigen (PSA) was retrospectively performed and demonstrated that continued monitoring of PSA levels could detect prostatic cancer many years earlier than usual clinical measures could.

---

[1] It is estimated that approximately one-third of the women enrolled in the hormone replacement therapy trial will have had a hysterectomy and therefore will not undergo the endometrial biopsy.

The Nun Study

The Nun Study is a longitudinal study of aging and Alzheimer's disease funded by the NIA. The Nun Study is based at the University of Kentucky, Sanders-Brown Center on Aging. A total of 678 women between the ages of 75 and 103 were drawn from the School Sisters of Notre Dame religious congregation. Each participant is annually assessed on her cognitive and physical function, and a brief medical exam is performed and a blood sample taken. Investigators have full access to each participant's archival and medical records. Each study participant has also agreed to donate her brain at death for further scientific study.

Bogalusa Heart Study

The Bogalusa Heart Study, ongoing since 1972, is the longest and most detailed study of children in the world. The Bogalusa Heart Study is an NIH-sponsored Specialized Center of Research (SCOR) at Louisiana State University Medical Center, run by a multidisciplinary team of anthropologists, biochemists, cardi-ologists, epidemiologists, geneticists, nurses, nutritionists, psychologists, soci-ologists, and statisticians. The study seeks to understand the environmental and hereditary aspects of early coronary artery disease, essential hypertension and cardiovascular risk factors in African-American and Caucasian children in the semirural community of Bogalusa, Louisiana. In addition, 160 substudies have been conducted, including special studies on socioeconomic evaluations, blood pressure, lipid levels, genetics, exercise, heart murmurs, and pathology. Knowledge gained in the Bogalusa Heart Study has been applied to develop, test, and evaluate methods for cardiovascular risk intervention.

The Bogalusa Heart Study has conducted cross-sectional and longitudinal observations on more than 14,000 children and young adults. For example, a post–high school study currently follows subjects until 38 years of age. Blood samples have been sent to Boston, Baltimore, Sweden, and Finland for special analysis. More than 632 publications, three textbooks, and numerous mono-graphs have been produced using samples and data from the Bogalusa Heart Study.

National Health and Nutrition Examination Survey

Since 1960, the National Center for Health Statistics (NCHS) of the CDC has conducted seven health examination surveys of the population of the United States: the National Health Examination Surveys (NHES) Cycles 1, 2 and 3, the National Health and Nutrition Examination Surveys (NHANES) I, II and III, and the Hispanic Health and Nutrition Examination Survey (HHANES). The surveys are designed to assess the health and nutritional status of children and adults in the United States periodically through interviews and direct physical examinations. The surveys employ interviews to answer questions about demographics, socioeconomic status, dietary habits, health-related issues, and physical and dental examinations, which include physiologic assessments and laboratory tests. Blood samples are collected as part of the physiologic assessments and placed in storage banks after laboratory tests are completed.

Cumulatively, the health examination surveys have analyzed and banked samples from more than 85,000 participants. The most recent survey, NHANES III, conducted between 1988 and 1994, performed laboratory tests on approximately 30,000 people of all races aged 2 months and older from 81 counties in 26 states. Some of the 30 topics investigated in the NHANES III included high blood pressure, high cholesterol, obesity, secondhand smoking, lung disease, osteoporosis, HIV/AIDS, hepatitis, helicobacter pylori, immunization status, diabetes, allergies, growth and development, anemia, dietary intake (including fats), antioxidants, and nutritional blood measures. The NHANES I analyzed blood and urine samples from 23,808 study participants, and NHANES II analyzed 20,322 samples. The HHANES was a one-time survey conducted from 1982 to 1984 that provided data on 11,653 people of Hispanic origin.

National Institute of Allergy and Infectious Disease- Division of AIDS

The Division of the Acquired Immunodeficiency Syndrome (DAIDS) was formed in 1986 to address the national needs of the cause and spread of HIV/AIDS. The mission of DAIDS is to increase basic knowledge of the pathogenesis, natural history, and transmission of HIV disease and to promote research in the detection, treatment, and prevention of the disease. DAIDS supports a number of longitudinal as well as clinical trials programs in the epidemiologic, therapeutic, and vaccine/prevention research as described below and in Chapter Two.

Individually and collectively, these studies have amassed a wealth of data that provides detailed information on the natural history and clinical and laboratory course of HIV disease in various populations. Specific fluids and tissues collected from the various studies include peripheral blood, mononuclear cells, serum, plasma, semen, saliva, vaginal washings, urine, placenta, and autopsy samples. These samples together with the huge database to which they are linked provide a rich resource for multidisciplinary investigations to scientists.

The Multicenter AIDS Cohort Study and the San Francisco Men's Health Study. The Multicenter AIDS Cohort Study (MACS) and the San Francisco Men's Health Study, awarded in 1983 by DAIDS, is a longitudinal study of HIV infection in approximately 5,000 homosexual and bisexual men. The goals of the study are to provide an appropriate epidemiological basis for laboratory-based studies of HIV pathogenesis; to study the changing natural history of HIV infection; to define subgroups of HIV-infected individuals with unique HIV-related outcomes; and to identify individuals who remain HIV seronegative despite ongoing or prior high-risk sexual activity. Clinical specimens are collected on a regular basis (every six months) and include cells, serum, plasma, and tissue (including lymph node tissue and tissue collected at autopsy).

The Women and Infants Transmission Study. The Women and Infants Transmission Study (WITS) is a collaborative, multisite, longitudinal study of U.S. women with HIV infection and their offspring. As of September 1995, more than 1,200 women and almost 1,000 infants have been enrolled in the study. The goals of the study are to determine maternal cofactors related to maternal-infant HIV transmissions; to ascertain the timing of perinatal transmission and the risk factors for ante- versus intrapartum transmission; to evaluate HIV disease progression among both pregnant and nonpregnant HIV-positive women; to assess the natural history of infants born to HIV-positive women and determine factors affecting disease progression; and to establish effective means for early diagnosis of HIV infection in infants. Adult specimens collected during the study include blood, urine, and genital samples. Pediatric specimens include blood and urine.

The Women's Interagency HIV Study. The Women's Interagency HIV Study (WIHS), awarded in 1993, is a collaborative, multisite, longitudinal study established to investigate the impact of HIV infection on U.S. women. As of September 1995, more than 2,300 women were enrolled. The goals of the study are to describe the spectrum and course of clinical manifestations of HIV infection in women; to describe the pattern of immune markers in HIV-infected women; to investigate factors that may delay or accelerate HIV-induced immune dysfunction and specific HIV-related conditions; and to study the length of survival and quality of life of women living with HIV infection. Specimens routinely collected from study participants include blood, oral/pharyngeal swabs, urine, vaginal and cervical swabs, and cervicovaginal lavage fluids.

Framingham Heart Study

Since 1948, the federal government has followed a representative sample of 5,209 adults in Framingham, Massachusetts. These people have been tracked using standardized biennial cardiovascular examinations, daily surveillance of hospital admissions, death information, and information from physicians and other sources outside the clinic. The goal has been to study the epidemiology of cardiovascular diseases and to learn the circumstances under which they arise, evolve, and terminate fatally in the general population. The study is also designed to differentiate those who develop cardiovascular diseases from those who remain disease-free over a longer period of time.

Physicians' Health Study

The Physicians' Health Study, conducted at Brigham and Women's Hospital in Massachusetts since 1982, is a randomized, double-blind, placebo-controlled trial studying the role of aspirin and beta-carotene in decreasing risks of cardiovascular disease and cancer. The study has been conducted entirely by mail among 22,701 U.S. male physicians between the ages of 40 and 84 years of age. In addition, blood specimens have been collected from each participant.

The Physicians' Health Study II will evaluate the effects of beta-carotene, vitamin E, vitamin C, and multivitamin supplements on the prevention of cancer, especially prostate cancer in a randomized, double-blind, placebo-controlled trial. Fifteen thousand U.S. male physicians will be enrolled in this study.

Nurses' Health Study

The Nurses' Health Study began in 1976 at the Harvard School of Public Health. Since then, 117,000 nurses have entered the study. The study was designed to serve as a prospective follow-up study to examine a possible relationship between oral contraceptive use and breast cancer. Follow-up questionnaires have been mailed to participants every two years, and blood specimens were collected at the time of enrollment. Extensive details of lifestyle practices have been collected for each participant. The Nurses' Health Study has been a part of many studies investigating the relation between use of hormones, diet, exercise, and other lifestyle practices as related to the development of various illnesses, including diabetes, breast cancer, and colon cancer.

Health Professionals Follow-Up Study

The Health Professionals Follow-Up Study was initiated in 1986 at Harvard University. More than 51,000 male health professionals aged 40 to 75 years were followed, and blood specimens were obtained from each of the participants. This study has been the basis for several prospective studies investigating factors that are potentially important in the development of prostate cancer, colon cancer, colorectal adenoma, cardiovascular disease, chronic dental disease, kidney disease, multiple sclerosis, and Parkinson's disease.

MRFIT Study

The Multiple Risk Factor Intervention Trial (MRFIT) was a cardiovascular disease intervention trial. MRFIT began by screening 361,662 males between the ages of 35 and 57 from 1973 to 1975. More than 12,000 men were then enrolled in the intervention trial. Lifestyle data were collected from each participant as well as blood serum samples. Data have been used in studies measuring the relationship between such factors as serum cholesterol, smoking, hypertension, and stress with the development of cardiovascular disease.

Women's Health Study

The Women's Health Study, conducted at Brigham and Women's Hospital, will evaluate the balance of benefits and risks of low-dose aspirin and vitamin E in reducing the risks for cardiovascular disease and cancer in women. The study population will consist of 40,000 U.S. female health professionals age 45 and older.

RESEARCH THAT SIMULTANEOUSLY CREATES TISSUE COLLECTIONS OR CONTRIBUTES TO A TISSUE BANK

Most research projects that use human tissue obtain specimens from pathology laboratories or existing tissue banks. However, some research studies require unique samples and must collect specialized tissue. Therefore, some research will create tissue collections and may end up contributing these samples to an established tissue bank for storage. Several examples of research that simultaneously creates tissue collections or contributes to a tissue bank are described below.

National Institute of Child Health and Human Development

NICHD performs and supports several research projects in pregnancy, delivery, and child development–related issues that involve collection and storage of tissue samples. To fulfill its needs for storage, monitoring and distribution of existing and yet-to-be-collected specimens, the NICHD contracts with commercial enterprises. For example, the Maternal Fetal Network Project, conducted by the Pregnancy and Perinatology Branch of NICHD, has contracted with Biotech Research Laboratory to establish a repository that will contain frozen plasma and sera samples from patients studied in several clinical protocols. This repository is a valuable source of biological markers for the study of preterm births and preeclampsia. In addition, two NICHD-funded research studies, the Diabetes in Early Pregnancy Study (DIEP) and a Longitudinal Study of Fetal Growth and Perinatal Outcome, have contracted with Biomedical Research, Inc., to provide storage, monitoring, and distribution of serum samples. Both studies involved collecting multiple blood samples throughout the course of the study. Biomedical Research, Inc., also provided storage, monitoring, and distribution of serum, plasma, and urine from a double-blind, randomized, clinical trial of supplemental calcium for the prevention of preeclampsia during pregnancy. Five clinical centers, enrolling 4,500 women over a two-year period, contributed samples from study participants at baseline, early and late in the third trimester of pregnancy, and at the time of diagnosis of preeclampsia.

Prostate Cancer Intervention Versus Observation Trial

The primary objective of the Prostate Cancer Intervention Versus Observation Trial is to determine which of these two strategies is superior for the management of clinically localized prostate cancer: radical prostatectomy with early intervention or expectant management with reservation of therapy for palliative treatment. The VA Medical Center in Minneapolis, Minnesota, is the central location of the study, and the project is supported by the Department of Veterans Affairs. One thousand patients from 80 medical centers with clinically localized prostate cancer who are under 75 years of age and potential candidates for radical prostatectomy will be included in the study. A central laboratory will examine tissue specimen samples for confirmation of histopathologic diagnosis of prostate cancer. Also, a centralized serum bank will be established for PSA assays and future studies.

Smoking Cessation Program for Patients Enrolled in SPORE Projects

The VA Medical Center in Denver, Colorado, is conducting a study to understand the epidemiologic finding that former smokers remain at elevated risk for many years after cessation of smoking. The study is supported by the Department of Veterans Affairs. The aims of the study include assessing the degree and time course of reversion of preneoplastic markers to normal after smoking cessation in smokers who are at high risk for lung cancer and to characterize individuals who do not show reversion of these markers to normal after smoking cessation. A bank of sputum cytology samples will concurrently be established for a cohort of high-risk subjects. Samples from high-risk subjects before and after smoking cessation will be used for rapid pilot testing of new lung cancer markers.

Genetics of Familial Polycystic Ovary Syndrome

Researchers at the Milton S. Hershey Medical Center in Pennsylvania are studying polycystic ovary syndrome (PCOS) to find a genetic marker that would be useful in identifying women at risk for developing PCOS prior to the onset of complications. The study will include a few large, three-generation kindreds of PCOS to reduce genetic heterogeneity. A DNA bank of complete PCOS pedigrees is being assembled for genetic studies. A normative database will be established for age, weight, and ethnicity matched controls. Previously identified kindreds of familial PCOS will be phenotyped for clinical, biometric, and biochemical abnormalities. All available pedigree members—male and female—will be phenotyped. By identifying women at risk for PCOS, medical resources could be focused on preventing complications.

Molecular Basis of Split Hand/Split Foot Malformation

The University of North Carolina at Chapel Hill is characterizing the molecular defect responsible for split hand/split foot (SHSF) malformation, a human developmental disorder that results in abnormal hands and feet. A repository of cell lines from individuals with SHSF and related malformations is being established. This resource will facilitate cloning of the SHSF gene as well as future investigations of genotype-phenotype relationships in SHSF. SHSF pedigrees will also be analyzed. Isolation of the SHSF gene will provide an opportunity to investigate the molecular basis of pattern formation in the human limb.

Molecular Epidemiology of Breast Cancer

Case Western Reserve University in Cleveland, Ohio, is pursuing a study to understand the molecular epidemiology of breast cancer entitled "Establishment of an at-risk cohort and methods to improve the collection and use of risk." The study is funded by the Department of the Army and will specifically investigate molecular markers and their interaction with other epidemiologic risk factors toward identification of relative risk factors for breast cancer development in Caucasian and African-American women with benign breast disease. More than 5,000 women are expected to be followed to yield an estimated 250 breast cancer cases. Benign breast disease and cancerous tissue samples will be archived in a specimen bank. A questionnaire will be developed to identify risk factors and will be used to construct an exposure index for lifetime exposure to sex hormones.

Human Conceptual Tissue: Characterization for Transplantation

The Puget Sound Blood Center of Seattle, Washington, is committed to determining the availability and suitability of embryonic tissue for transplantation research and therapy. In this project, investigators will focus on development and assessment of protocols for the collection, processing, and cryopreservation of embryonic tissue and will also characterize hematopoietic stem cells derived from embryonic fetal liver. This project is supported by the National Institute of Child Health and Human Development. Three institutions participate in this project (the Central Laboratory for Human Embryology, the Northwest Tissue Center, and the Fred Hutchinson Cancer Research Center), and together they have formed the Northwest Fetal Tissue Program. For more than 30 years, the Central Laboratory for Human Embryology has collected and processed more than 15,000 embryos and fetuses. The other groups have expertise in storage and cryopreservation of tissue and stem cell replacement therapy research.

Epidemiology of EBV-Defined Hodgkin's Disease

The Northern California Cancer Center is conducting a study to explore the epidemiology of subtypes of Hodgkin's disease defined by Epstein-Barr virus. The study will collect specimens archived between 1990 and 1995 from Hodgkin's disease cases reported to the California Cancer Registry; apply standard techniques to classify each case as Epstein-Barr virus–positive or –negative; calculate risks of Epstein-Barr virus–positive and –negative Hodgkin's disease for multiple variables; calculate incidence rates of Epstein-Barr virus–positive and –negative Hodgkin's disease; and bank tumor specimens for future testing. It is expected that tumor specimens will be requested for more than 2,500 subjects.

Therapy and Biological Correlations of Soft Tissue Sarcoma

Fifty percent of patients who undergo surgery in conjunction with radiotherapy do not have successful survival rates, usually due to pulmonary metastases. These metastases can only be marginally controlled by toxic chemotherapy agents if they are not resectable. Other problems surrounding the understanding and successful treatment of soft tissue sarcomas include different and noninterconvertible staging systems, a lack of information about molecular determinants of sarcoma proliferation and metastasis, and long-term clinical trials due to the rarity of the disease resulting in slow drug production. This project at the University of Texas M.D. Anderson Cancer Center, supported by the NCI, will focus on these obstacles in the area of soft tissue sarcomas. A bioresource facility has been established that contains a tissue bank, short-term culture explants and cell lines, and paraffin-embedded tissue blocks.

Lifetime Alcohol Exposure and Breast Cancer Risk

The Department of the Army funds a population-based, case-control study to investigate the relationship between alcohol exposure and the risk of breast cancer at the State University of New York at Buffalo. African-American and Caucasian women, aged 35 to 79, both pre- and postmenopausal will be selected. Matched controls will be randomly selected. A specimen bank will be created to store biological samples for future studies.

Prospective Randomized Study of Adjuvant Chemotherapy Versus Vinorelbine and Cisplatin in Completely Resected NSCLC with Companion Tumor Marker Evaluation

This phase III study will be conducted at the VA Medical Center in East Orange, New Jersey, and is supported by the Department of Veterans Affairs. The study compares the overall survival between completely resected patients with T2NO, T1-2NI non–small cell lung cancer (NSCLC) who have received either adjuvant chemotherapy with vinorelbine and cisplatin or observation alone. A comprehensive tumor bank will be established and linked to a clinical database. These tissue specimens will be used for further study of molecular markers in resected NSCLC.

Case-Control Study of Hodgkin's Disease in Children

This is an ongoing study at the University of Pittsburgh supported by the NCI to investigate the epidemiologic, virologic, and genetic components of the rare cases of Hodgkin's disease in children. Previously, epidemiologic data had been gathered from 300 cases and 484 controls by telephone interviews. The project will be expanded to 415 cases and 675 controls. Tissue specimens will be collected from all 415 cases for virologic assays and to create a biologic specimen bank for future studies.

Markers for Differential Diagnosis and Virulence of Prostate Cancer

A project on molecular markers for differential diagnosis and virulence of prostate cancer is being conducted at the VA Medical Center in Seattle, Washington, and supported by the Department of Veterans Affairs. This study will focus on the development of reagents and immunoassays for various serum forms of PSA, to determine whether CD44 and specific isoforms enable prostatic cells to metastasize to specific sites and to construct cDNA libraries from a prostate cancer xenograft model. A human tumor/sera bank will also be established for multiple other projects.

The Role of IL-1 Cytokines in Colorectal Cancer

The VA Medical Center in Pittsburgh, Pennsylvania, is conducting a project to delineate gene products that are inappropriately expressed in colorectal tumors that may affect clinical outcome. A second goal of the project is to identify gene products essential to tumor cell proliferation and may serve as therapeutic targets. A tumor bank has been established of frozen tumors and polyps from more than 200 cases. A database contains clinical and pathological findings for each stored specimen.

Markers for Malignant Progression in Prostate Cancer

A study investigating molecular prognostic markers to assist in clinical management and classification of patients into clinical trials is being conducted at Georgetown University. The goal of the study is to identify molecular markers and activated oncogenes that indicate poor prognosis in prostate cancer. The study will actively accrue freshly frozen surgical material to a prostate tissue bank. The tumor bank will maintain demographic information and pathology records and blocks.

Pulmonary Hypertension- Mechanisms and Family Registry

This project will be conducted at Vanderbilt University Hospital in Nashville, Tennessee, and is supported by NHLBI. The goals of the project will be to investigate the basic mechanisms of primary pulmonary hypertension and to establish a registry and database of familial primary pulmonary hypertension pedigrees to determine the mode of inheritance. A tissue bank will be set up for DNA samples and transformed lymphocytes from families and patients with primary pulmonary hypertension. These samples will be made available to investigators both locally and nationwide.

Blood Test to Predict Prognosis in Patients with Gynecologic Cancer: Plasma Assay of GLB and GLB:TIMP-1 Complexes

The Department of Veterans Affairs supports this study at the VA Medical Center in Northport, New York. It is believed that the production and activation of enzymes known as gelatinases (GLA and GLB) are essential components for tumor metastasis. An ELISA test has been developed to measure the concentrations of GLB and its complexes in plasma from patients with cancer. It has been demonstrated that these enzymes are increased in plasma from patients with gynecologic and colorectal cancer. The goals of this study are to establish a plasma bank from patients with gynecologic cancers (ovarian, cervical, uterine, vaginal), to measure the plasma concentration of GLB and its complexes and to determine whether the plasma concentrations of GLB and its complexes can be uses as a prognostic and response factor to different treatment regimens.

AIDS-Malignancy Clinical Trials Consortium

The University of Southern California AIDS-Malignancy Clinical Trials Consortium (AM-CTC) helps design, develop, and conduct collaborative, innovative phase I and II clinical trials, employing novel agents and approaches in patients with various AIDS-related malignancies. In addition, the AM-CTC provides tumor tissue and other relevant biologic materials, derived from patients accrued into clinical trials, to the NCI-funded Tissue and Biological Fluids Bank of HIV Associated Malignancies. Since 1987, the AIDS Clinical Trials Group (ACTG) has accrued more than 470 patients onto various AIDS-malignancy protocols. The University of Southern California AIDS Malignancy Program has been actively engaged in phase I and II trials related to HIV-related cancers, with participation in 45 such studies, resulting in 17 publications, and 30 published abstracts.

Pancreatic Cancer Case-Control Study in San Francisco

This population-based, case-control study in men and women will examine the hypotheses linking adenocarcinoma of the exocrine pancreas and detailed occupational history and chemical exposures. This study is supported by the NCI. One thousand cases and 1,150 controls will be interviewed during a 3.5-year period. The study is based at the University of California, San Francisco, and will include participants from six San Francisco Bay area counties. Blood samples for genetic investigations will be drawn, and cells samples will be frozen in the Irwin Memorial Blood Bank. Whole-blood specimens will also be stored for future genetic and biomarker studies.

Exogenous Toxicants and Genetic Susceptibility in Amyotrophic Lateral Sclerosis

Stanford University is investigating the role of environmental toxicants and genetic susceptibility factors in the etiology of Amyotrophic Lateral Sclerosis (ALS) by conducting a case-control study of 175 incident ALS and 550 age- and gender-comparable control subjects. All 175 ALS cases and a subset of 350 control subjects will undergo measurement of bone lead stores using x-ray fluorescence and will have a venous blood sample drawn for copper-zinc superoxide dismutase (SOD1) enzyme genotyping and DNA banking. The collection of detailed information regarding the duration and timing of environmental exposures will enable the evaluation of dose response trends and estimation of latent periods between putative exposure and the development of ALS. It is hoped that the proposed study will advance knowledge of neurotoxic and endogenous susceptibility factors important in the etiology of ALS.

National Institute of Allergy and Infectious Disease- Division of AIDS

DAIDS was created in 1986 to address the national research needs created by the cause and spread of HIV/AIDS. Several clinical research trials groups are sponsored by DAIDS and have collectively amassed a large number of specimens that are available for research.

The HIV Network for Prevention Trials. The HIV Network for Prevention Trials (HIVNET), established in 1994, is a network of clinical sites to conduct HIV vaccine efficacy trials and prevention trials in higher-risk populations. HIVNET consists of five contracts supported by DAIDS: the domestic HIV/AIDS vaccine efficacy trials, the international HIV/AIDS vaccine efficacy trials, a statistical and data coordinating center, a specialized laboratory testing center, and a specimen repository. As of September 1995, more than 3,600 volunteers had participated in HIVNET. Specimens collected from HIVNET trials are routinely sent to a central laboratory for testing. HIVNET specimens include serum, plasma, peripheral mononuclear cells, genital tract specimens, and saliva. The availability of specimens depends on the type of specimen requested.

The Pediatric AIDS Clinical Trials Group. The Pediatric AIDS Clinical Trials Group (PACTG), awarded in 1987, is a multicenter clinical trials network. The goals of this study group are to support the development and implementation of phase I, II, and III studies designed to test and optimize therapies to prevent and treat HIV infection and its sequelae in infants, children, and adolescents; to conduct studies throughout the United States at more than 50 pediatric AIDS Clinical Trials Units; and to collaborate closely with the adult ACTG studies. Specimens collected from PACTG trials included serum, plasma, peripheral mononuclear cells, culture supernatants, lymph node biopsies, tissues, urine, and other body fluids.

The Adult AIDS Clinical Trials Group. The Adult AIDS Clinical Trials Group (Adult ACTG), established in 1987, is a consortium of 30 clinical trial research groups. The goals of the adult ACTG are to evaluate innovative therapeutic strategies and interventions to control HIV infection and complications in adults; to facilitate rapid translation of basic research into clinical research and practice; and to provide a flexible resource for state-of-the-art, multi-disciplinary clinical trials. To date, more than 35,000 adult volunteers at all stages of the disease have enrolled. Specimens collected during the clinical trials include serum, plasma, peripheral mononuclear cells, culture super-natants, lymph node biopsies, tissues, urine, and other bodily fluids.

The AIDS Vaccine Evaluation Group. The AIDS Vaccine Evaluation Group (AVEG), consists of six AIDS Vaccine Evaluation Units that evaluate candidate AIDS vaccines in phase I and II clinical trials for safety and immunogenicity. As of October 1995, more than 1,800 volunteers had enrolled in AVEG trials. Specimens collected during clinical trials include serum, plasma, peripheral mononuclear cells, genital tract secretions, saliva, and tears. The availability of specimens depends of the type of specimen requested.

The Division of AIDS Treatment Research Initiative. The Division of AIDS Treatment Research Initiative (DATRI), established in 1991, conducts phase I and II studies of therapies for HIV and associated diseases. The DATRI Network performs small, focused studies and substudies of protocols conducted by other extramural programs. Clinical specimens will vary according to protocol and include serum, plasma, cells and cultured cells, and supernatant from PBMC and plasma HIV cultures.

Chapter Six

PATHOLOGY SPECIMENS

A large number of tissues are collected for diagnostic or therapeutic reasons. These tissues are usually sent to a clinical, diagnostic or pathology laboratory for examination. These laboratories may be located at GME teaching institutions, physicians' offices, community hospitals, or independent laboratories. These tissues may sometimes be used for research, educational, and quality-control purposes, though the vast majority are not. Most patients sign a general consent stating that after completion of any diagnostic tests, some of the sample can be saved/used for research purposes.

To be accredited, laboratories must keep pathological specimens for a minimum amount of time. The Clinical Laboratory Improvement Amendments of 1988 (CLIA) set forth the conditions that laboratories must meet to be certified to perform testing on human specimens. CLIA stipulates that laboratories must retain cytology slides for a minimum of five years, histopathology slides for a minimum or 10 years, and paraffin blocks for a minimum of two years (CLIA, 1996). In addition, some states have regulations that require retention of pathology specimens for longer than the time specified in the CLIA regulations. For example, New York, which has some of the most stringent regulations, requires that laboratories retain abnormal cytology slides for 10 years, cytology slides with no abnormalities for five years, and histopathology slides and paraffin blocks for 20 years. Once the regulated length of time for storage is met, institutions may continue to store pathology specimens based on the room they have for storage, the philosophy of the institution, and several other variables.

PATHOLOGY DEPARTMENTS AT GRADUATE MEDICAL EDUCATION TEACHING INSTITUTIONS

Medical education in the United States can be divided into three major phases. The first phase, medical school, provides instruction in the sciences that underlie medical practice and in the application of those sciences to health care. In 1997, there were 125 medical schools in the United States (including three in

Puerto Rico) (American Medical Association, 1997). The second phase, graduate medical education (GME), prepares physicians for independent practice in a medical specialty. GME programs, usually called residency programs, are based in hospitals or other health-care institutions, some of which have and some of which lack formal relationships with medical schools. GME teaching institutions include medical schools, U.S. armed forces hospitals, VA medical centers, the Public Health Service, state, county, and city hospitals, nonprofit institutions, and health maintenance organizations. In 1997, 1,687 accredited GME teaching institutions operated in the United States (including 22 programs in Puerto Rico) (American Medical Association, 1997). Continuing medical education (CME), the third phase of medical education, updates medical professionals' education throughout their careers.

Collectively, pathology departments at GME teaching institutions constitute the largest and oldest stores of tissue samples in the United States. Two techniques were used to estimate the total number of cases accessioned per year at all GME institutions and the number of tissues stored at each institution. The first estimate used information found in the American Medical Association's Graduate Medical Education Directory 1997–1998 about residency programs in pathology at GME institutions (American Medical Association, 1997). However, information was not available about all pathology specialties. Therefore, a second estimate was made from information obtained from several chairs of pathology departments attending a meeting of the Universities Associated for Research and Education in Pathology (UAREP), hosted by the Federation of American Societies for Experimental Biology (FASEB).[1]

The number of pathology residency positions at a GME teaching institution is determined by the caseload of the pathology department. The Graduate Medical Education Directory stipulates that programs should have a sufficient number of cases to ensure that residents have a broad exposure to both common and unusual conditions and that the number of resident positions requested by an institution not exceed the educational resources available in a program (American Medical Association, 1997). The actual number of GME programs and residency positions in 1995–1996, and the number of programs and proposed residency positions for 1997–1998 are shown in Table 6.1. Table 6.2 shows the recommended number and types of cases/specimens residents should examine during their training in anatomic and clinical pathology, dermatopathology, forensic pathology, neuropathology, or pediatric pathology.

---

[1]Medical schools represented at the UAREP meeting included those at the University of Pittsburgh, Johns Hopkins University, University of Minnesota, Robert Wood Johnson Medical School, University of Kansas, Case Western Reserve University, University of Pennsylvania, University of Iowa, Northwestern University, Thomas Jefferson University, and Memorial Sloan-Kettering.

This information was not available for the specialties of cytopathology, chemical pathology, hematology, immunopathology, or microbiology.

An analysis was performed to estimate the total number of cases accessioned per year at all GME teaching institutions in the pathology specialties of anatomic and clinical pathology, dermatopathology, forensic pathology, neuropathology, and pediatric pathology. This calculation was based on several criteria: the number of GME pathology programs in each specialty; the number of resident positions open in these programs for the academic year; the recommended number of cases per program to meet the training requirements of the residents; and the duration of the program in years. Table 6.3 contains data for the academic year 1995–1996, and Table 6.4 contains data for 1997–1998. Information on the recommended number of cases per resident was not available for all pathology specialties. However, an effort was made to obtain information on the average number of cases/specimens accessioned per institution each year for cytopathology and hematopathology, the two other pathology specialties in Table 6.1 with large numbers of residency positions.

Of the pathologic specialties, anatomic and clinical pathology, cytopathology and hematopathology specimens probably account for the largest collection of tissues. For the academic year 1996–1997, there were 180 anatomic and clinical pathology programs with 2,675 residents (see Table 6.1). To have enough cases to fulfill the educational needs of their residents, institutions would have had to

Table 6.1

GME Pathology Programs and Residency Positions

Pathology Specialty	1996–1997[a]		1997–1998[b]	
	Number of Programs	Number of Residents	Number of Programs	Number of Residents
Anatomic and Clinical	180	2,675	180	2,656
Cytopathology	68	74	68	101
Chemical Pathology	7	4	7	6
Dermatopathology	41	54	41	72
Forensic Pathology	39	47	39	73
Hematopathology	54	51	54	119
Immunopathology	9	6	9	12
Microbiology	9	5	9	9
Neuropathology	47	37	47	66
Pediatric Pathology	20	12	20	28
Total	474	2,965	474	3,142

[a]Graduate Medical Education, 1997.

[b]American Medical Association, 1997.

accession more than five million total cases/specimens, an average of 28,050 cases/specimens per program (Table 6.3). Similarly, in 1997–1998, the 180 anatomic and clinical pathology programs with 2,656 residency positions would have to accession more than five million total cases/specimens, an average of 27,851 cases/specimens per program (Table 6.4). Some of the specimens collected by anatomic and clinical pathology may be referred to in another specialty, such as dermatopathology, neuropathology, or immunopathology, and given a separate accession number within that specialty. Therefore, some specimens listed in Tables 6.3 and 6.4, especially for dermatopathology and neuropathology, may also have been accounted for as anatomic and clinical pathology cases. Forensic pathology cases are accessioned separately from the other specialties. It is recommended that forensic pathology programs conduct approximately 500 medicolegal autopsies per year and approximately 300 additional autopsies for each additional residency position. Therefore, forensic pathology programs would have had to conduct 21,900 autopsies[2] in 1996–1997, and 29,700 in 1997–1998 to provide enough cases for resident training.

Table 6.2

Recommended Specimens for Pathology Residency Programs

Pathology Specialty	Recommended Cases/Specimens per Resident
Anatomic and Clinical	≥75 autopsies ≥2,000 surgical pathology specimens ≥1,500 cytologic specimens ≥200 intraoperative consultations (frozen sections)
Dermatopathology	≥5,000 new accessions
Forensic Pathology[a]	250–350 autopsies
Neuropathology[b]	≥50 neuromuscular biopsy specimens
Pediatric Pathology	≥40 pediatric autopsies ≥2,000 pediatric surgical pathology specimens ≥50 intraoperative consultations (frozen sections/ smears)

SOURCE: American Medical Association, 1997.

[a]In addition to the 250–350 autopsies recommended for residents in Forensic Pathology, it is recommended that forensic pathology programs conduct approximately 500 medicolegal autopsies per year and approximately 300 additional autopsies for each additional residency position requested.

[b]In addition to the minimum of 50 neuromuscular biopsy specimens recommended for residents in neuropathology, it is recommended that neuropathology programs conduct at least 200 necropsies and examine at least 100 neurosurgical specimens per year.

---

[2]A single autopsy case may generate several slides and paraffin blocks.

Table 6.3

Specimens and Autopsy Cases Accessioned in 1996- 1997

Pathology Specialty	Number of Specimens[a] per Year	Number of Programs	Number of Specimens[a] per Program per Year
Anatomic and Clinical[b]	5,049,063	180	28,050
Dermatopathology	270,000	41	6,585
Forensic Pathology	21,900	39	562
Neuropathology	14,100	47	300
Pediatric Pathology	25,080	20	1,254

[a]Includes autopsy cases.

[b]Anatomic and Clinical Pathology programs range in length from 18–24 months. Therefore, the number of specimens per year represents the number of programs multiplied by the number of residents (Table 6.2) divided by two years (24 months) as a minimum estimate.

Table 6.4

Specimens and Autopsy Cases Accessioned in 1997- 1998

Pathology Specialty	Number of Specimens[a] per Year	Number of Programs	Number of Specimens[a] per Program per Year
Anatomic and Clinical[b]	5,013,200	180	27,851
Dermatopathology	360,000	41	8,780
Forensic Pathology	29,700	39	762
Neuropathology	14,100	47	300
Pediatric Pathology	58,520	20	2,926

[a]Includes autopsy cases.

[b]Anatomic and Clinical Pathology programs range in length from 18–24 months. Therefore, the number of specimens per year represents the number of programs multiplied by the number of residents (Table 6.2) divided by two years (24 months) as a minimum estimate.

In some institutions, pediatric pathology cases may go directly to the pediatric pathology department. However, in some institutions, they may first be accessioned in anatomic and clinical pathology. The 12 residents in pediatric pathology programs in 1996–1997 would have conducted 480 pediatric autopsies and examined 24,000 pediatric surgical pathology specimens and 600 intraoperative consultations (frozen sections, smears). To support 28 pediatric pathology resident positions in 1997–1998, a total of 58,520 specimens and autopsy cases would have to be accessioned. A conservative estimate is that an average of approximately 30,000 anatomic and clinical, forensic, and pediatric pathology and autopsy cases are seen per GME teaching institution each year.

An estimate of the number of cases/specimens accessioned in cytopathology and hematopathology programs was obtained by averaging the number of cases/specimens reported on various GME teaching institutions' Web sites. Table 6.5 shows information obtained for cytopathology, and Table 6.6 shows information about hematopathology. Cytopathology programs accession an average of approximately 50,000 cytology specimens per year (range of 14,000 to 100,000 cases/specimens). Hematopathology programs accession an average of 750 bone marrow aspirations and biopsies and resections of lymph nodes and related tissue.

As an independent method to estimate the average number of pathology cases accessioned per institution each year, chairs of pathology departments attending the UAREP meeting were asked several questions about the pathology

Table 6.5

Cytopathology Programs

Program	Specimens per Year
University of North Carolina	>24,000
Emory University	65,500
University of Wisconsin	100,000
University of Michigan	47,500
Georgetown University	14,000
Total	251,000
Average	50,200

Table 6.6

Hematopathology Programs

Program	Specimens per Year[a]
NYU Medical Center	750
Emory University	1,000
University of Michigan	500
Total	2,250
Average	750

[a]The College of American Pathologists Minimum Guidelines for the Retention of Laboratory Records and Materials recommends a retention time of 10 years for bone marrow specimens but only 24 hours for serum, cerebral spinal fluid, and other body fluids and seven days for peripheral blood and body fluid smears (http://www.cap.org). Therefore, specimens recorded here represent the number of bone marrow aspirations and biopsies and resections of lymph nodes and related tissue accessioned at each institution listed.

departments at their institutions. Information was obtained about the size of their institution, the number of cases accessioned per year, the age of the oldest tissues archived, how long the tissue samples are stored, what identifying information is kept with the tissues, and who has access to the samples. The medical schools represented had facilities that ranged from 250 beds to approximately 2,000 beds and accessioned from approximately 10,000 to approximately 60,000 cases per year. The medical schools accessioned an average of 40 cases per bed with a range of 20–60 cases per bed. Most of the pathology departments stored tissue samples indefinitely, with the oldest tissues archived anywhere from 20 years old to more than 100 years old. Stored specimens are either labeled with a pathology accession number linked to the patient's medical record or labeled directly with the patient's name and medical record number. People who have access to the specimens include the pathologists, researchers, other physicians, and anyone with a court order. Each institution accessions an average of approximately 30,000 cases per year, with approximately 3.8 million total cases accessioned per year at all 125 medical schools in the United States.

DNA DIAGNOSTIC LABORATORIES

GeneTests

GeneTests is an online national directory of DNA diagnostic laboratories. GeneTests seeks to promote the appropriate use of genetic counseling and testing in patient care. GeneTests maintains a comprehensive list of clinical service and research laboratories performing inherited disease–specific clinical molecular genetic testing for single-gene and contiguous-gene disorders. GeneTests is funded by the National Library of Medicine and the Maternal and Child Health Bureau and administered through the Children's Hospital Regional Center in Seattle, Washington. In January 1994, 148 laboratories were listed in GeneTests—131 in the United States, 16 in Canada, and one in Mexico (McEwen and Reilly, 1995). One hundred and thirty-seven of the labs were academically based or within government agencies, and 11 were commercial laboratories (McEwen and Reilly, 1995).

In a 1994 survey of GeneTests (formerly known as HELIX) DNA diagnostic laboratories, 90 percent of the respondents (93 of 148 (63 percent) laboratories surveyed responded) stated that they banked DNA (McEwen and Reilly, 1995). DNA banks ranged in size from fewer than 100 to more than 1,000 samples in storage (McEwen and Reilly, 1995). Most laboratories banked DNA as a service to referring physicians or for individuals and families at risk for a particular genetic disorder, for such research purposes as gene mapping, and as a service to clinical, forensic, or research laboratories (McEwen and Reilly, 1995). More than half of the respondents stated that their laboratories had released samples to researchers after stripping the samples of identifiers (McEwen and Reilly, 1995).

CLINICAL SERVICE AND DIAGNOSTIC LABORATORIES

The majority of clinical service and diagnostic laboratories are not associated with GME teaching institutions. These include laboratories within physicians' offices or community hospitals and independent laboratories. In 1991, approximately 640,000 clinical laboratories and other facilities performed laboratory tests on human specimens (Department of Health and Human Services, 1991). The number of tissues stored at these laboratories varies greatly, but the minimum storage time is determined by CLIA and state regulations and College of American Pathologists guidelines.

CENTERS FOR DISEASE CONTROL AND PREVENTION INSTITUTES

The Centers for Disease Control and Prevention (CDC), in Atlanta, Georgia, is an agency of the Department of Health and Human Services. The CDC's mission is to promote health and quality of life by preventing and controlling disease, injury, and disability. The CDC is made up of six centers, one institute, and four offices.[3] Several centers have stored tissue samples, including the National Center for Environmental Health and the National Center for Infectious Disease.

National Center for Environmental Health

The National Center for Environmental Health (NCEH) is involved in several areas of research, including biomonitoring, breast cancer–related projects, and genetic research. The NCEH has also prepared DNA specimens from approximately 8,000 NHANES (describe in Chapter Five) participants to be used by researchers around the country. In 1996, eight breast cancer–related projects collected more than 3,500 serum samples for analysis in such studies as "Breast Cancer Among Women Exposed to Polybrominated Biphenyl" and "Breast Cancer Among Native Alaskan Women Exposed to Organochlorines."

---

[3]The institute, offices, and centers within the CDC are the National Center for Chronic Disease Prevention and Health Promotion, the National Center for Environmental Health, the National Center for Health Statistics, the National Center for HIV, STD, and TB Prevention, the National Center for Infectious Diseases, the National Center for Injury Prevention and Control, the National Institute for Occupational Safety and Health, the Epidemiology Program Office, the Office of Global Health, the Public Health Practice Program Office, and the office of Genetics and Disease Prevention.

National Center for Infectious Diseases

The National Center for Infectious Diseases (NCID) plans, directs, and coordinates a national program to improve the identification, investigation, diagnosis, prevention, and control of infectious diseases. The NCID also maintains several tissue banks. The NCID's Scientific Resources Program maintains a bank of serum specimens of epidemiological and special significance to CDC's research and diagnostic activities. The NCID is also responsible for the integrity, security, and maintenance of a computer inventoried serum bank consisting of 250,000 aliquots of serum from 100,000 Alaskan Natives.

Chapter Seven

STATE SCREENING LABORATORIES
AND FORENSIC DNA BANKS

The collection of blood specimens for disease testing, paternity testing, or forensic testing has grown enormously in the last quarter of the twentieth century. As biomedical technology advances, more and more testing will be performed on smaller and smaller sample sizes. Although tissue samples may be collected for a specific purpose, it is not unlikely for them to be used for other reasons. These large collections of human tissue samples have been a matter of concern for privacy advocates.

NEWBORN SCREENING LABORATORIES

Archives of newborn screening cards for inborn errors of metabolism (Guthrie cards) represent an enormous source of banked DNA. Guthrie cards are used to screen newborns for several diseases, including congenital hypothyroidism, phenylketonuria, galactosemia, hemoglobinopathies (e.g., sickle-cell anemia), biotinidase deficiency, homocystinuria, Maple Syrup Urine disease, and cystic fibrosis. These newborn screening tests utilize bacterial inhibition assays and automated enzymatic methods. However, as new genetic screening tests are developed, and the Human Genome Project discovers new disease-related genes, it is likely that newborn screening tests may become DNA-based. In addition, scientific interest in using Guthrie cards for populationwide genetic epidemiological studies has grown, given the stability of DNA in dried blood and the ability to analyze the DNA in these samples (McEwen and Reilly, 1994).

A 1994 survey of all newborn-screening programs in all 50 states, the District of Columbia, Puerto Rico, and the Virgin Islands revealed that the majority of laboratories have accumulated less than 500,000 Guthrie cards over the years, seven have amassed more than 500,000, four reported collections of between one million and five million cards, and one reported a collection of six million (McEwen and Reilly, 1994). The number of cards collected over a one-year period ranged from <10,000 in four labs to >500,000 in two especially populous states (McEwen and Reilly, 1994). For example, better than 99 percent of the 550,000 children born each year in California are tested for three genetic conditions (Reilly, 1992).

The trend in most states is to save Guthrie cards for longer and longer periods of time. Eleven laboratories indicated that their state departments of public health have issued written regulations on the retention of Guthrie cards, while 29 stated that their laboratories have internal written policies on this matter (McEwen and Reilly, 1994). Forty of the state newborn screening laboratories retain all the Guthrie cards they receive through their newborn-screening programs, including those cards that test negative, at least for a short period of time (McEwen and Reilly, 1994). Twenty-three laboratories indicated that they keep their cards for a year or less, 10 plan to keep their cards for one to five years, 13 will keep them for longer than five years, three save all their cards for 20–25 years, and four plan to keep their cards indefinitely (McEwen and Reilly, 1994). Thirteen other respondents discard their cards within several weeks or months (McEwen and Reilly, 1994).

Guthrie cards contain identifying information, such as the mother's name and address, hospital of birth, baby's medical records number, and the name and address of the baby's doctor. The conditions under which Guthrie cards are stored vary from state to state. Some store the cards in boxes at room temperature, some keep them in boxes or folders in a freezer, refrigerator, or climate-controlled room, some keep them in boxes or folders in a basement or warehouse, and some keep them in a cabinet either in folders or biohazard bags (McEwen and Reilly, 1994). Fourteen state laboratories periodically check the condition of their stored cards (McEwen and Reilly, 1994).

All states participate in some form of newborn screening, but few have issued regulations that explicitly define the scope of permissible use of Guthrie card samples (Andrews, 1995). Seven state departments of public health have issued written regulations on third-party access to Guthrie cards, and 10 of the laboratories have internal written policies on this matter (McEwen and Reilly, 1994). Over a five-year period, 28 laboratories estimated that they had received either no requests or fewer than six third-party requests, seven received six to 20 requests, two received 21–100 requests, and one, from a very large state, received more than 100 requests (McEwen and Reilly, 1994).

FORENSIC DNA BANKS

In 1989, the Virginia Division of Forensic Science was the first state laboratory to offer DNA analyses to law enforcement agencies and the first to create a DNA databank of previously convicted sex offenders. By November 1997, 48 states had established forensic DNA data banks of convicted criminals, especially violent sex offenders and other violent felons (Finn, 1997). The two states without forensic DNA banks, Vermont and Rhode Island, are planning legislation to create them (Finn, 1997). In addition, the Federal Bureau of Investigation (FBI) is exploring ways to create a forensic DNA bank for the District of Columbia (Finn, 1997).

The DNA Identification Act of 1994 (Pub. L. No. 103-322, 1994 HR 3355, 108 Stat. 1796, §210304), a federal law enacted in fall 1994 as part of the Omnibus Crime Control Law, created a national oversight committee to develop guidelines for DNA forensics and established a five-year, $40 million grant program to assist state and local crime laboratories in developing or improving forensic DNA testing capabilities. The DNA Identification Act also formally authorized the FBI to establish Combined DNA Index System (CODIS) for law enforcement identification purposes (TWGDAM, 1989). CODIS is a national computer network containing DNA profiles of convicted offenders, unknown suspects, and population samples (used for statistical purposes only). Using CODIS, federal, state, and local law enforcement agencies can compare DNA profiles from crime scenes to DNA profiles of felons in the CODIS database.

CODIS provides a framework for storing, maintaining, tracking, and searching DNA specimen information. Currently, CODIS has been implemented in 45 states, encompassing greater than 90 percent of the U.S. population. Each CODIS database consists of three distinct indexes—casework, convicted offender, and population. The casework and convicted felon indexes are used to search for matching DNA profiles of specimens from crime scenes.

In addition to collecting specimens from sex offenders and violent felons, a number of states require samples from juvenile offenders, nonviolent felons, such as drug or white collar offenders, and those convicted of misdemeanors (McEwen, 1997). South Dakota requires samples from people merely arrested (not convicted) of a sex offense (Finn, 1997), with several other states considering similar bills (McEwen, 1997). There is also a proposal to establish a federal DNA databank that would include profiles from people convicted in federal or military courts of offenses similar to those covered by most state laws (McEwen, 1997).

Convicted offenders are required to provide blood, or in some cases saliva, either at sentencing or before release from prison (McEwen, 1997). Some states also require samples from people already incarcerated before laws' effective dates (McEwen, 1997). The DNA from these samples is analyzed for its unique identification characteristics. Nationwide, samples from about 380,000 offenders have been collected, mostly in Virginia and California, and about 116,000 samples (30 percent) have been analyzed (McEwen, 1997). These DNA identification profiles are stored, along with the samples themselves, to help identify suspects by matching biological evidence found at crime scenes to state DNA databases.

DNA profiles prepared from these samples have already proven valuable for tracing biological material found at crime scenes to felons with prior convictions. By February 1997, forensic DNA databanks had achieved more than 200 cold hits linking serial rape cases or identifying suspects by matching DNA extracted from biological evidence found at a crime scene to that of a known offender whose DNA profile was in the databank. For example, Minnesota's DNA data bank was used to tie the same individual to 18 separate assaults (McEwen, 1997).

DNA testing has the power to not only implicate an individual in a crime, but also to exonerate an apparently innocent individual. Recently, a Texas man who had served 12 years in prison for rape was pardoned after he was cleared of the crime by DNA tests (Holmes, 1997). Semen samples kept from 1985 were tested and failed to match his DNA. Several private laboratories have been established in the last 20 years that offer DNA testing services, such as paternity testing, parentage testing, forensic DNA analysis, and expert witness services.

Chapter Eight

CRYOPRESERVATION FACILITIES/STORAGE BANKS

The concept of storing human tissue for future use by either the donor or an anonymous person is a concept that arose during the last half of the twentieth century. Organ transplants were the first surgical procedure to be performed that involved the placement of a person's organs into the body of another to replace a diseased organ. Organs, though, cannot be stored for long periods and thus must be transplanted within hours of removal from the donor (as described in Chapter Nine). Today, sperm and embryos can be frozen and thawed and still be viable for artificial insemination procedures or implantation. The newest type of human tissue storage for future use is the storage of umbilical cord blood.

SPERM, OVUM, AND EMBRYO BANKS

Artificial insemination or donor insemination (DI) is a procedure to achieve conception when natural methods have failed. Sperm may be donated by a woman's husband or by another donor. The first successful artificial insemination was performed in 1790, and donor insemination was first successfully performed in 1884. Both procedures used fresh semen samples. The concept of storing human sperm for long-term use was not realized until the 1970s when the first commercial sperm banks opened, although the first successful donor insemination using frozen sperm occurred in 1953. It was not until 1985 that frozen sperm became the standard for donor insemination. The public recognition of the dangers of AIDS posed a new threat to the use of fresh semen samples, and several organizations began to discourage the use of fresh semen and recommended that only frozen sperm that had been quarantined for a minimum of six months be used for DI. In 1995, there were more than 280 fertility clinics in the United States and 57,000 assisted reproductive technology (ART) cycles were performed. Most of these cycles used the couple's own egg and sperm to produce embryos.

A few of the major cryobanks and fertility clinics that store human embryos, sperm, and/or oocytes are described below. A more comprehensive list of cryopreservation facilities and fertility clinics with storage services can be found in Appendix I.

California Cryobank, Inc.

California Cryobank, Inc., founded in 1977, is one of the largest full-service sperm banks. The California Cryobank provides physicians and their patients a comprehensive resource for semen cryopreservation and specialized reproductive services. It is accredited by the American Association of Tissue Banks, and licensed by the state departments of health in California, Maryland, Massachusetts, and New York. The California Cryobank offers the following services: the freezing and storing of anonymous human sperm for use in artificial insemination; long-term semen storage for men facing the possibility of sterilization, reduction in fertility potential, or genetic damage due to vasectomy, chemotherapy, radiation therapy, and high-risk occupational exposures; long-term storage of preimplantation embryos; and andrology laboratory services, such as semen analysis, fertility testing, sperm washing, and sex selection. California Cryobank's staff includes physician medical directors, genetic counselors, donor matching counselors, and technical staff.

The California Cryobank's donor catalog currently contains more than 200 donors, who agree to leave semen donations at least once per week for nine to 12 months. Donors must complete a donor profile that contains a detailed, three-generation medical and genetic history that includes information about the donor's parents, siblings, grandparents, aunts, and uncles. This donor profile is provided to the patient. Donor profiles also include personal information, such as the donor's religion, physical characteristics, favorite sports, favorite pets, SAT scores, educational background, and work experience. All donors undergo genetic testing for sickle-cell anemia, Tay-Sachs disease, and cystic fibrosis carrier status. Donors are also tested for infectious diseases, including hepatitis B and C, CMV, sexually transmitted diseases, and HIV/AIDS. All semen specimens are quarantined for at least six months, during which donors are retested every three months for these infectious diseases. Both donor and patient records are kept indefinitely.

California Cryobank has written standard operating procedures pertaining to the storage and maintenance of reproductive tissue. These procedures require a designated secure area for storage tanks that is locked at all times and has limited access, extensive external and internal security systems, personnel to monitor the liquid nitrogen level of each storage tank daily, and complete records of all tissues stored and all activities pertaining to the stored tissues.

Quality-control measures include racially color-coded donor specimens and an electronic identification system to identify donors prior to each deposit.

Cryobanks International, Inc.

Cryobanks International, Inc. (CI), is a "Cryocenter" that unites parallel technologies of freezing autologous blood, semen, and umbilical cord blood within one facility. One of the services of CI is to provide anonymous donor semen to couples and individuals.

Genetics & IVF Institute

The Genetics & IVF Institute (GIVF), founded in 1984, is one of the largest, fully integrated providers of infertility treatment and genetics services. The GIVF has a main facility in Fairfax, Virginia, and a second facility in Gaithersburg, Maryland. In the Fairfax facility, the GIVF provides medical diagnosis and treatment; genetic and reproductive laboratory testing, including paternity testing; and cryobank services.

The GIVF's Cryopreservation Division, established in 1986, produced the first frozen human embryo twins in the United States. The cryobank services include embryo cryopreservation and storage, sperm banking, and human ovarian tissue cryopreservation. The institute's embryo cryopreservation program currently freezes 2,300 embryos annually and has produced more than 250 pregnancies.

Fairfax Cryobank

The Fairfax Cryobank, a sperm bank, was established in 1986 to provide patients at GIVF with anonymous frozen donor semen. Fairfax Cryobank was the first sperm bank in the United States to test for genetic carriers of BRCA1, Gaucher's disease and Canavan's disease in Jewish donors and cystic fibrosis, alpha-1 antitrypsin, and HIV by polymerase chain reaction (PCR) in all donors. Fairfax Cryobank also tests for Tay-Sachs in Jewish donors, thalassemia in Asian, Middle Eastern, and Mediterranean donors, and sickle-cell anemia and other hemoglobinopathies in African-American donors. Fairfax Cryobank is one of the largest human sperm banks in the country and has provided donor specimens throughout the United States and abroad.

UMBILICAL CORD BLOOD BANKS

Stem cells—progenitor cells, which produce all other blood cells—are used to treat patients with blood diseases, patients with certain genetic disorders, and patients receiving chemotherapy and/or radiation treatment for cancer. Until scientists discovered that umbilical cord blood contained hematopoietic stem cells, the only known source of stem cells was bone marrow. The retrieval of bone marrow, though, is invasive, may be painful, requires general anesthesia, and is expensive. In contrast, retrieval of umbilical cord blood is noninvasive, painless, and generally takes only a few minutes to complete. After a baby is delivered and the umbilical cord is cut, blood is withdrawn from the umbilical cord and placenta with a syringe and then cryogenically stored. In addition, bone marrow is difficult to match between donor and recipient, while cord blood is compatible with more people. Cord blood transplants also have a lower incidence of graft versus host disease (GVHD) and are less likely to transmit infectious diseases.

In 1988, the first successful human cord blood transplant was performed in a child with Fanconi's anemia using cord blood from a sibling (Gluckman et al., 1989). Since then, over 500 autologous and allogeneic umbilical cord blood transplants have been performed worldwide, with the majority done in the past two to three years (Perdahl-Wallace, 1997). Approximately two-thirds of the cord blood transplants have been performed for malignant conditions, including acute lymphocytic leukemia, acute myelocytic leukemia, chronic myelogenous leukemia, and neuroblastoma (Wagner et al., 1995). The other one-third have been for a variety of genetic disorders, including Hurler's syndrome and Hunter's syndrome, adrenoleukodystrophy, osteopetrosis, severe aplastic anemia, severe combined immunodeficiency, and hemoglobinopathies, such as beta thalassemia and sickle-cell anemia (Wagner et al., 1995; Wagner et al., 1996). The majority of transplants have been in children, although a few adults have been transplanted as well.

Under an NIH-sponsored program, cord blood is now being collected and stored at several large banks around the United States, including the New York Blood Center, Duke University, Indiana University, and the University of Minnesota. The International Cord Blood Registry, maintained by the University of Minnesota, matches requests for allogeneic transplants with cord blood banks. In addition, the NHLBI is sponsoring a five-year, $30 million study to show whether cord blood transplantation is a safe and effective alternative to bone marrow transplantation. The collection and storage centers for this study are at Children's Hospital of Orange County, Duke University, and the University of California at Los Angeles.

In the last few years, privately owned companies have also begun offering umbilical cord blood banking services to individuals and families. When dealing with private storage companies, users pay a one-time fee for the collection, testing, and freezing of the blood. An annual fee is charged for storing the blood in liquid nitrogen. The stored cord blood may be withdrawn if illness occurs later. In contrast, when parents donate their baby's cord blood to a public bank, they generally pay no fees, but they give up all rights to the sample to help build the public supply of cord blood for use in transplantation and research. Even though umbilical cord blood banking has become popular, the Working Group on Ethical Issues in Umbilical Cord Blood recently concluded that "until additional data are obtained regarding safety and efficacy, umbilical cord blood banking and use ought to be considered an investigational technology rather than a proven treatment" (Sugarman et al., 1997).

Public Donor Umbilical Cord Blood Banks

American Cord Blood Program. The American Cord Blood Program, located at the University of Massachusetts Medical Center, is the first nonprofit umbilical cord blood bank in New England. The American Cord Blood Program, partially funded through a grant from the National Children's Cancer Society, is only the eighth public donor cord blood bank in the world. To date, the American Cord Blood Program is the only academic health center in the country with a comprehensive program of cord blood collection, banking, transplantation, and research.

The first donation of cord blood was made on January 2, 1997. Since then, the American Cord Blood Program has collected more than 1,000 cord bloods and hopes to get 10,000 cord blood donations by 2007. Expectant mothers are asked to contact the program between 28 and 30 weeks of pregnancy to become donors. The mother is given a kit to bring to the hospital on the day of delivery. However, hospitals keep spare kits on hand. Blood collected from the umbilical cord vein is sent to the University of Massachusetts to be typed, frozen, and stored at the American Cord Blood Bank until a match is found.

The research component of this program is conducted at the University of Massachusetts. Research continues in several areas, including investigating the ways cord blood cells divide, studying engraftment of transplanted cord blood cells in mice, and developing other applications of cord blood transplantation, such as for gene therapy.

Chicago Community Cord Blood Bank. The goal of the Chicago Community Cord Blood Bank (CCCBB) is to collect units of cord blood, test them for infectious diseases, identify the protein markers (HLA molecules) required for matching the cord blood to patients, and store them for future transplantation into patients with cancer or other life-threatening diseases. The CCCBB, at University of Chicago Children's Hospital, is a community resource dedicated to providing units of cord blood for stem cell transplantation and medical research. The CCCBB is currently supported by grants and private donations, which cover the cost of collection, testing, and storage (approximately $1,000 per cord blood unit).

The CCCBB has been in operation for about two years and has collected approximately 300 cord blood units. The majority of cord blood is donated for use in unrelated allogeneic transplants. However, less than 10 percent of cord bloods stored at CCCBB are family donations for use in related transplants for family members at risk or in need of stem cell transplants. There is no charge to donors for the processing and storage of cord blood units.

Expectant mothers who donate their baby's cord blood are asked to consent to providing medical, ethnic, and related information, donating the cord blood to the cord blood bank for transplantation and/or research, allowing blood to be drawn from the mother for tests, including HIV testing, and granting permission to track the newborn's medical history for up to one year. No blood is drawn from the baby for the cord blood bank. A minimum of 50 cc of cord blood is necessary for use in transplantation. However, approximately 10 percent of cord blood collections yield less than 50 cc and are used for research or quality-control purposes.

International Cord Blood Foundation. The International Cord Blood Foundation, established in 1995, is a nonprofit, public bank that stores umbilical cord blood for use in unrelated, anonymous transplants. The foundation holds the policy that before prospective donors decide to donate, they must be fully educated about the importance of cord blood, its potential uses, and the options available (family banking versus donation to a public bank versus disposal). Donors are required to supply a variety of personal information to ensure the safety of the donated cord blood. The foundation keeps all information confidential and does not provide it in a form allowing personal identification unless compelled to by legal order or other lawful authority.

The International Cord Blood Foundation does supply cord blood for research purposes to universities and other institutions. Cord blood is normally used for research when it is not suitable for transplantation, such as when not enough blood is collected from the placenta or not enough nucleated cells are in the specimen. The possibility that the donated cord blood may be used for research is mentioned in the informed consent that donors sign.

New York Blood Center. The New York Blood Center's (NYBC) placental blood program, established in 1993, was the nation's first program for storing umbilical cord blood for allogeneic transplantation. The NYBC placental blood program currently has an inventory of approximately 7,000 units of frozen umbilical cord blood (Torloni, 1997). The NYBC placental blood program is a nonprofit storage program funded by the NHLBI.

St. Louis Cord Blood Bank. The St. Louis Cord Blood Bank at Cardinal Glennon Children's Hospital/St. Louis University is a public donor bank, not a private storage bank. In cooperation with other cord blood banks, the St. Louis Cord Blood Bank serves as a worldwide resource for children in need of stem cell transplants. The banking program includes community and donor education, cord blood collection, processing in the cord blood laboratory, release of the cord blood product, and evaluation of transplant outcomes. As of April 1997, more than 1,800 banked and fully characterized cord blood units were available at the St. Louis Cord Blood Bank.

Puget Sound Blood Center Cord Blood Bank. The Puget Sound Blood Center has recently established the Cord Blood Bank program. It is the only cord blood bank in the state of Washington and will be used by patients around the world. The Cord Blood Bank will seek 400 donations this year from donor mothers who deliver at Swedish Medical Center in Seattle and Kapiolani Medical Center for Women and Children in Honolulu.

Related Umbilical Cord Blood Bank for Hemoglobinopathy Patients. The Related Umbilical Cord Blood Bank for Hemoglobinopathy Patients at Children's Hospital Oakland in California is supported by the NHLBI. Umbilical cord blood has been recognized as a source of hematopoietic stem cells and has been used in transplants in patients with hemoglobinopathies. The purpose of this project is to store umbilical cord blood for genetically related patients with hemoglobinopathies for transplants. The bank will serve as a resource to hemoglobinopathy centers. The bank will also serve as a research resource for evaluation of the role of umbilical cord blood transplantation in patients with hemoglobinopathies.

Private Umbilical Cord Blood Banks

Cord Blood Registry. Cord Blood Registry, in partnership with the University of Arizona School of Medicine, provides state-of-the-art facilities for the collection, processing, and long-term cryogenic storage of umbilical cord blood for parents who wish to store their newborns' cord blood. Cord Blood Registry also established the Designated Transplant Program to allow qualified families in imminent need of stem cell transplants to store their newborns' cord blood free of charge. Umbilical cord blood stem cells banked at the Cord Blood Registry have been used for both related and unrelated transplants.

Families not in imminent need of stem cell transplants store umbilical cord blood with Cord Blood Registry on the remote chances that the child it came from or another family member may need a stem cell transplant in the future. Cord Blood Registry requires mothers to sign an informed consent at least 30 days prior to collection of the cord blood. Each client who privately stores cord blood receives a certificate of legal ownership for their deposit. When samples are not suitable for transplantation due to small sample size or shortage of nucleated cells in the sample, the family is given a refund and recontacted as to the disposition of the sample. Families are given the choice to donate the cord blood for use in research or to request that the sample be disposed of.

Cord Blood Registry also has programs in education and research. In 1996, more than a million pieces of educational material were distributed to the public and medical communities through Cord Blood Registry's national network of Medical Education Specialists and Cord Blood Educators outreach programs. Cord Blood Registry also sponsors continuing medical education programs led by cord blood experts in major institutions across the country. As a founding member of the International Cord Blood Foundation (see "Public Donor Umbilical Cord Blood Banks"), Cord Blood Registry provides substantial support to help fund the foundation's educational and public health initiatives and assists with the National Marrow Donor Program to educate the transplant and research communities. In addition, Cord Blood Registry makes a $200 donation from each privately banked cord blood to the foundation to help in the collection and processing of cord blood. Combined, the Cord Blood Registry and the International Cord Blood Foundation have collected more than 8,000 umbilical cord blood units.

New England Cord Blood Bank. The New England Cord Blood Bank, Inc., is part of the New England Cryogenic Center, Inc., a private cryogenic laboratory. Since its establishment in June 1997, New England Cord Blood Bank has stored more than 200 units of umbilical cord blood for use in autologous transplants or for related transplants in family members. New England Cord Blood Bank does not store cord blood for unrelated allogeneic transplants. If a family decides to terminate their storage agreement at New England Cord Blood Bank, the sample can be donated to a public bank to help others in need of stem cell transplants.

Cryobanks International, Inc. Cryobanks International, Inc. (CI), also cryogenically stores human umbilical cord blood in its multiservice complex. The purpose of CI's bank is to develop a registry of donated umbilical cord blood for transplantation, to provide affordable personal umbilical cord blood storage, to provide storage for vital blood tissues, and to provide anonymous donor semen to couples and individuals.

Reproductive Genetics Institute. For almost a decade, the Reproductive Genetics Institute (RGI) has provided state-of-the-art genetics services, including genetic counseling, prenatal diagnosis, DNA diagnosis, forensic identification, paternity testing, IVF, and preimplantation genetic diagnosis. Established in 1990, RGI is a private enterprise and was one of the first to provide chorionic villus sampling in the United States. Scientists at RGI are involved in basic research in human genomics, experimental embryology, and cell genetics. The Cell and Tissue Bank, including an umbilical Cord Blood Bank, contains living biological samples available for research and practical application. Types of the cells/tissues available include 107 diploid cell strains from embryos of different gestational ages, chromosomally abnormal cell strains obtained from spontaneously aborted embryos and abnormal embryos, cell strains from skin fibroblasts of patients with single gene disorders, more than 100 human umbilical cord blood samples, hundreds of sperm samples, and dozens of donor oocytes.

Viacord. Viacord, Inc., is a medical service company that provides private family cord blood banking. Physicians refer expectant families to Viacord to have their newborn's cord blood processed and banked for another immediate family member in need or at risk of needing a stem cell transplant arising from a known malignancy, genetic blood disorder, or other relevant disease. In addition, families with no apparent need or risk also bank cord blood at Viacord, although the chances of needing it within the family are relatively small.

Viacord's comprehensive cord blood banking services include everything from training of the obstetrician and labor and delivery staff on proper collection procedures to testing and typing, cryopreservation, and storage of umbilical cord blood. Expectant mothers and their physicians complete an extensive health questionnaire and appropriate informed consents. The expectant mother is tested for infectious diseases once during the third trimester and again at delivery. The cord blood is tested for the number of stem cells (CD34-positive cells) and bacterial and fungal contamination and typed for blood type (ABO and Rh) and histocompatibility (HLA-A and HLA-B). The testing and typing results are provided to the referring physician.

A number of insurance companies have begun to pay for Viacord's services when the newborn's sibling or parent is in need of or has significant risk of needing a stem cell transplant. Blue Cross Blue Shield, Aetna Health Plan, Prucare, and even some state Medicaid providers have paid in full for collection, processing and storage of cord blood for these families.

ORGAN BANKS/BLOOD BANKS

ORGAN BANKS

Organ and tissue banks recover, process, store, and distribute human organs, bone, and tissue for transplantation. Donations are made from people who agree to donate upon their death. A single organ and tissue donor can save or improve the lives of 40–50 people: by donating up to seven vital organs, two eyes for corneal transplants, and bone and soft tissue to benefit 30–40 others. Some organ and tissue banks may also have tissue available for educational and research purposes. However, the demand for organs, bone, and tissue usually exceeds the supply. Therefore, only organs and tissues not suitable for transplantation are available for research. A few organ and tissue banks are described below, and Appendix H contains a partial list of organ and tissue banks in the United States.

Eye banks have been one of the fastest growing types of tissue banks in the latter half of this century. The first eye bank opened in 1946 in New York City and was operated by Dr. R. Townly Paton, who is known as the father of modern eye banking. Currently, almost 100 banks operate in the United States. The advancing technologies in corneal transplant have stimulated the growth of eye banks, and, as with other organs, the demand for transplant tissue is greater than the supply. In 1997, more than 85,000 eye donations (corneas or whole globes) were reported from U.S. Eye Banks (Eye Bank Association, 1998). In 1997, more than 43,000 eye donations were used for corneal transplants and more than 21,000 were used in research (Eye Bank Association, 1998). More than 550,000 cornea transplants have been performed since 1961 with a 90 percent success rate in restoring sight (Eye Bank Association, 1998).

Many of the nonprofit eye banks are funded by local Lions Clubs. Several eye banks are briefly described below that donate tissue for research purposes as well as transplantation procedures. For a more complete list, refer to Appendix H for a state-by-state listing of organ banks.

Northwest Tissue Center

A division of the Puget Sound Blood Center, the Northwest Tissue Center provides musculoskeletal and cardiovascular tissue for transplantation in Washington, Alaska, Montana, and Idaho. Established in 1988, the center is the region's only full-service, nonprofit tissue bank. Each year tissue is provided for more than 4,000 allografts. The donor's medical history and circumstances surrounding the donor's death are gathered from the health-care provider. The donors are screened for infectious, neurological, and autoimmune diseases as well as cancer and drug abuse. Additional information is provided by family members. Laboratory testing for HIV, HTLV-I and-II, hepatitis B and C, and syphilis ensures the safety of the donated tissue. The process is confidential, and the recipients do not know from whom the tissue was received.

New England Organ Bank

The New England Organ Bank (NEOB), a collaborative enterprise of six Boston hospitals started in 1968, is the oldest independent organ bank in the United States. Currently it is a federally designated organ procurement organization for all parts of the six New England states, including thirteen transplant centers with the capability to perform all types of organ and tissue transplantation. Through the United Network for Organ Sharing (UNOS), the NEOB provides organs for transplant outside of New England when a compatible recipient cannot be found in New England. NEOB Tissue Services began recovering bone and other musculoskeletal tissues for orthopedic surgeons in 1988. All tissues procured are collected, processed, tested for infectious diseases, stored, and distributed according to the Standards for Tissue Banking of the American Association of Tissue Banks.

Rochester Eye and Human Parts Bank, Inc.

The Rochester Eye and Human Parts Bank, Inc., was originally founded as the Rochester Eye Bank and Research Society in 1952 by the Downtown Lions Club. In 1968, the eye bank expanded to include the collection of all organs and tissues and adopted its current name. The bank currently procures, processes, preserves, and distributes eyes, skin, and cardiovascular and musculoskeletal tissues for transplant, research, and medical education.

Old Dominion Eye Bank

The first eye bank in Virginia was established in 1956 through the Medical College of Virginia. In 1962, the eye bank was reorganized and came under the direction of the Old Dominion Eye Foundation, Inc., a nonprofit organization, and the Old Dominion Eye Bank (ODEB). ODEB is supported by multiple Lions Clubs. ODEB serves as a receiving, processing, research, and distribution center for donated eye tissue. ODEB coordinates events from the time of the donor's death to the transplantation of the eye tissue. ODEB provides human eye tissue for corneal transplants, ophthalmic research, and educational training.

Utah Lions Eye Bank

The mission of the Utah Lions Eye Bank is to procure, test, evaluate, and distribute quality eye tissue for transplantation and research. The eye bank accepts donor tissue from donors of any race, religion, or age. Tissue specimens are supplied to researchers investigating macular degeneration and retinal cell transplantation at the John A. Moran Eye Center. Tissue may also be requested by physicians and other professionals for teaching, research, and development of new surgical techniques at the University School of Medicine.

Iowa Lions Eye Bank

The Iowa Lions Eye Bank in the Department of Ophthalmology and visual science at the University of Iowa was established in 1955. The eye bank is a nonprofit service committed to the restoration and preservation of sight through the collection, processing, and distribution of human ocular tissue for transplantation and research. Research areas include eye pathology, ocular melanoma, macular degeneration, and molecular ophthalmology. Tissue is first made available to Iowa surgeons for transplant. If it cannot be used in Iowa, it is then offered to other states and abroad. If the tissue is unsuitable for transplant, it is distributed to various research programs in the Department of Ophthalmology at the University of Iowa and to surgeons throughout the state. In 1995, the eye bank received 30 percent more eye donations than the previous year, 15 percent more in 1996, and 7 percent more in 1997. In 1995, the number of eyes distributed for transplant almost equaled the number distributed for research and training. In 1997, though, the number of donated eyes used for research was almost double the number used for transplants.

Kentucky Lions Eye Bank

The Kentucky Lions Eye Bank was founded in 1954. Its objective is to procure and distribute human donor eye tissue for transplant and ophthalmic research. In 1996, the eye bank had 204 eye donations. Tissue from eye donors aged 5–75 is suitable for transplantation if no problems are detected during the physical assessment or medical chart review of the donor. Tissue specimens that are distributed for research include whole eye, conjunctiva, lens iris/ciliary bodies, posterior poles (whole eye with the cornea removed), and cornea retina.

Central Florida Lions Eye and Tissue Bank, Inc.

The Central Florida Lions Eye and Tissue Bank, Inc. (CFLETB), was founded by a group of Tampa Lions in 1973. The eye and tissue bank is committed to the recovery, evaluation, and distribution of eye tissue for transplantation, research, and education. CFLETB has donated eye tissue to more than 20,000 individuals worldwide.

Mid-America Transplant Services

The Mid-America Transplant Services (MTS) is a fully accredited private, not-for-profit corporation designated by Medicare to coordinate the procurement of vital organs, eyes, bone, and soft tissue in hospitals throughout Missouri, southern Illinois, and northeastern Arkansas. Vital organs donated include heart, kidney, lung, liver, intestine, and pancreas. Tissues donated include eyes, long bones from the legs, heart valves, and tendons.

In 1995, MTS procured 318 vital organs from 97 local donors and imported another 147 vital organs. MTS also had 234 bone/soft tissue donors and 1,215 eye donors. All potential organ and tissue donors are carefully tested for cancer, infectious diseases, and AIDS before donation can proceed. Organ and tissue donation can proceed only after death has been declared and the next of kin has given consent. There is absolutely no cost to the donor family for organ or tissue donation.

The MTS Eye Banking Services recovers human eye tissue from recently deceased donors and then processes and preserves the tissue for distribution to ophthalmologists for corneal transplantation surgery. Donor eyes not suitable for transplantation may be given to researchers studying the causes and possible cures of blindness and to ophthalmology residency programs for education purposes, and for practicing ophthalmic surgery procedures. MTS also acts as a coordinating center for sharing of tissue among eye banks through its Tissue Sharing Services.

The eye tissue that MTS provides for research purposes includes whole eyes, posterior poles, lens, conjunctiva, retina, and choroid. Tissues can be preserved to meet the needs of individual researchers. Eyes from individuals with known eye diseases are especially valuable for study. In addition, MTS is involved in research to explore the possibility of retinal cell transplantation as a therapy for such diseases as retinitis pigmentosa and age-related macular degeneration. Donor tissue used for research on eye disease is extremely valuable to medical progress in treating blindness.

American Red Cross Tissue Services

The American Red Cross Tissue Services, established in 1984, collects, processes, and distributes human allograft tissue for use in transplantation. The Red Cross is one of the largest tissue collection-and-distribution organizations in the United States, supplying approximately one-quarter of the nation's tissues for transplantation. There are 17 tissue centers throughout the country and a national office in Washington, D.C. The American Red Cross Tissue Services distributes more than 70,000 units of tissue procured from more than 2,000 donors per year. For example, the Greater Northeast Area Tissue Services, the smallest of six Red Cross Tissue Centers, stores thousands of bone, skin, connective tissue, and heart valve samples from cadavers for transplantation, some research, and some education.

Tissue is obtained from deceased or surgical donors. Donors range in age from newborn to over 80. Tissue donors can sign a donor card but must make their wishes known to their families because the family's consent is required before tissues can be donated after death. All tissues are tested for diseases, such as AIDS, hepatitis, and syphilis.

The Red Cross distributes heart valves, skin, ligaments, tendons, bone, major blood vessels, and fascia, which covers muscles. These tissues are used in orthopedic, neurologic, ophthalmologic, plastic, cardiovascular, and oral reconstructive surgery for a wide range of medical procedures, such as salvaging limbs after tumor surgery, reconstructing hip and knee joints, replacing corneas, and correcting curvature of the spine. Tissue transplantation does not require the donor and the recipient to have the same blood type.

The Tissue Services Research program was established to provide research and development support to optimize human bone processing methods and to ensure the safety of American Red Cross allograft bone. It is a multidisciplinary effort with several departments, including Biochemistry, Coagulation Proteins, Experimental Pathology, Immunology, Molecular Biology, Plasma Derivatives, Platelet Biology, Product Development, Transmissible Diseases, and Virology. The Tissue Services Research program conducts in vivo and in vitro studies with human demineralized bone matrix to determine the bioactivity of various lots of bone. They are also developing a new bone delivery system for handling demineralized bone matrix during patient surgery. The Tissue Services Research program is also studying growth factors and viral inactivation.

Missouri Lions Eye Research Foundation

The Eye Research Foundation is located in Columbia, Missouri, and operates several different programs, including Eye Research, Operation of the Missouri Lions Eye Tissue Banks in three Missouri cities, Glaucoma Screening, Eyeglass Recycling, Amblyopia Screening, Indigent Patient Care, and Public Education. The foundation conducts research into eye diseases and disorders and ways to provide tissue of a higher quality for transplant purposes. In response to specific requests, the Foundation provides eye tissue for three corneal projects (University of Missouri, Kansas State University, and NIH), two glaucoma projects (St. Louis University, University of Nebraska), and two retinal cell transplant projects (Washington University, NIH).

BLOOD BANKS

During World War I, it was demonstrated that blood could be safely stored. Prior to World War I, a physician would screen a patient's friends and relatives until the proper type was found and then would bleed the donor and immediately transfuse the patient. Several discoveries in the early twentieth century, however, allowed for creation of blood banks today. In 1914, Luis Agote demonstrated that small, nontoxic quantities of sodium citrate could prevent coagulation of the blood, which led to the development of blood storage. In 1943, John Freeman Loutit and Patrick Loudon Mollison acidified the citrate and added dextrose, which allowed for the storage of red cells at 4°C for a period of 21 days. Further addition of adenine increased the storage time of blood in the liquid form. The first blood bank in the United States opened in 1937.

Whole blood can only be stored for a limited time, but various components of blood (red blood cells, platelets, albumin, and plasma fractions) can be frozen and stored for a year or longer. The cryoprotective agent glycerol protects red blood cells from destruction in freezing temperatures. Most blood donations, therefore, are separated and stored as components by blood banks. A single unit of blood can potentially serve the varying needs of five or more patients.

Blood banks exist in every state in the United States. As is common with organ banks, there are often shortages of specific types of blood, and blood drives are held to maintain existing stocks of all blood types. The American Association of Blood Banks (AABB) is an international organization of blood banks, transfusion and transplantation services, and those working in these groups—more than 2,200 institutions (community and hospital blood banks, hospital transfusion services, and laboratories) and 8,500 individuals are AABB members. The AABB also has an accreditation program that strives to improve the quality and safety of collecting, processing, testing, distributing, and administering blood and blood products.

America's Blood Centers (ABC), founded in 1962, is a national network of non-profit community blood centers. ABC members collect almost half (47 percent) of the U.S. blood supply at 450 donation sites in 46 states. ABC members are licensed and regulated by the U.S. Food and Drug Administration. Some of the nation's blood centers are briefly described below. For a more complete listing of U.S. blood centers, see Appendix H.

American Red Cross

The American Red Cross collected approximately 5.8 million blood donations in 1996. However, the Red Cross represents about half of all U.S. blood donations, so annually, about 12 million units of blood are donated in the United States. The American Red Cross usually maintains about a three-day supply of fresh blood as well as approximately 20,000 units of frozen blood at any one time. The American Red Cross also maintains the world's largest registry of frozen rare blood. Approximately 1,000 units of rare blood a year are supplied to recipients around the globe.

The Food and Drug Administration (FDA) requires the tracking of blood from "arm to arm," however this information is confidential and coded. Donors who test positive for HIV are notified and counseled. The consent form signed by donors asks if excess or expired blood may be used for research.

Fresh red blood cells have a shelf life of 21–42 days depending on the preservative used, and platelets have a shelf life of five days. Plasma can be stored frozen for one to five years, and frozen whole blood can be stored for at least 10 years. Platelets and red cells that expire are sold for research purposes. Researchers are informed that the samples have been found negative for all FDA required tests and only by special request may researchers be provided with the donor's age and gender. Plasma that cannot be transfused is used for making blood derivatives, such as Factor VIII for hemophiliacs, or for making diagnostic reagents. Nothing goes to waste.

Navy Blood Program

The Navy Blood Programs collects almost 150,000 units of blood per year. These units are stored for 35 days (like all blood). Also, 17,000 frozen units are kept on hand at all times. There is only a 6 percent expiration rate. A small amount of the blood that has passed the expiration date for transfusion may be used for research, but no specific program exists for supplying blood for research purposes. Any blood that tests positive for a disease is destroyed and not used for research purposes.

Community Blood Bank

The Community Blood Bank of Erie County, Pennsylvania, was founded in 1966 and was initially established as a donor recruitment agency. In 1985, the Community Blood Bank took on the responsibility of collection, processing, testing and distribution of blood and blood products. The Community Blood Bank exists as a nonprofit organization with the mission of providing a safe and adequate supply of voluntarily donated blood for patients in Erie County. The Community Blood Bank is the sole supplier of blood and blood products to Erie's six hospitals and to blood centers across the United States in need of emergency blood and blood products. The Community Blood Bank is an accredited AABB member.

Thomas Jefferson University Hospital Blood Bank

The Thomas Jefferson University Hospital Blood Bank is the oldest blood bank in the Philadelphia area. About 25 percent of all blood and blood components transfused at Jefferson are collected through the donor center (volunteer, autologous, and directed donors), and the remainder is obtained from the American Red Cross. The blood bank consists of four divisions: the Donor Center, Transfusion Unit, Pheresis Center, and Tissue Typing Laboratory. The blood bank is an accredited AABB member.

Blood Bank of Alaska, Inc.

The Blood Bank of Alaska, Inc., is a nonprofit organization established more than 25 years ago that serves 30 regional medical centers and hospitals. The blood bank offers services, including autologous donations, directed donations, platelet apheresis, allogeneic donations, and therapeutic phlebotomy. The Blood Bank of Alaska, Inc., is an AABB member.

New York Blood Center

The New York Blood Center (NYBC) has been in operation for more than 30 years. The NYBC is the nation's largest independent blood distribution and services organization, providing blood and blood products for more than one million transfusions annually, about 10 percent of the nation's blood supply. The NYBC serves more than 200 hospitals in New York, New Jersey, and Connecticut. The Lindsley F. Kimball Research Institute is housed in the NYBC and is a leading center for basic and applied research in hematology and transfusion medicine. The institute consists of 18 research laboratories committed to the study of blood and the prevention, treatment, and cure of bloodborne and blood-related diseases. NYBC also operates a Placental Cord Blood Program, and, since 1993, more than 500 transplants have been performed using cord blood provided by NYBC's Cord Blood Program. NYBC is a not-for-profit corporation and is an AABB member.

Puget Sound Blood Center

The Puget Sound Blood Center and Program was founded in 1944 and is the major resource for blood, tissue, and specialized services in the western Washington area. The Blood Center serves patients in more than 70 hospitals and clinics with blood services and provides tissue and transplantation support through the Northwest Tissue Center to 185 hospitals across the northwest United States. In 1997–1998, there were more than 170,000 volunteer blood donors. The Blood Program also maintains a research facility recognized internationally for advancements in transfusion and transplantation medicine.

Chapter Ten

CONCLUSIONS

Tissue collections vary considerably, ranging from formal repositories to the informal storage of blood or tissue specimens in a researcher's freezer. Appendix A reviews the sources of stored tissue samples described in this report. Archives of human tissue range in size from less than 200 to more than 92 million specimens. Appendix B provides estimates for the number of cases and specimens of stored tissue for each category of tissue collection and an estimate of the overall number of stored tissue samples in the United States. Conservatively, more than 307 million specimens from more than 178 million cases of stored tissue exist in the United States, accumulating at a rate of over 20 million per year.

The two largest tissue repositories in the world, the National Pathology Repository and the DNA Specimen Repository for Remains Identification, are housed in a single institution, the AFIP. These two repositories alone store more than 94 million specimens (Appendix A). The tissue repositories supported by NIH may not be as large as those at AFIP, but NIH is probably the largest funder of extramural tissue repositories, supplying more than $53 million in FY 1996. Finally, the pathology departments at GME teaching institutions collectively constitute the largest and oldest stores of tissue samples in the United States, with some specimens more than 100 years old. The tissue bank with the oldest samples in the world is the Egyptian Mummy Tissue Bank in Manchester, England, which contains mummy tissue dating back to 2686 B.C.

The vast majority of tissues were originally collected for diagnostic or therapeutic reasons. Three sources—the AFIP National Pathology Repository, GME teaching institution pathology departments, and Newborn Screening Laboratories—represent more than 265.5 million diagnostic and therapeutic specimens from more than 176 million cases. At the AFIP National Pathology Repository alone, more than 92 million pathologic specimens from more than 2.5 million cases are stored (Appendix A). Of the 1,687 GME Teaching Institutions with residency programs in cytopathology (68 institutions), hematology (54 institutions), and clinical and anatomic pathology (180 institutions), well over eight million cases are accessioned cumulatively per year. Pathology departments at GME teaching institutions without pathology residency programs also accession pathology specimens but most likely not at the same rate as institutions with pathology residency programs. Most GME teaching institutions retain pathology specimens indefinitely, with the oldest tissues anywhere from 20 years old to more than 100 years old. Therefore, at a rate of eight million cases a year for 20 years, conservatively more than 160 million cases are stored at GME teaching institutions with pathology residency programs with several million more stored at those without pathology residency programs. By 1994, the majority of Newborn Screening Laboratories had accumulated less than 500,000 Guthrie cards over the years, seven have amassed more than 500,000 (greater than 3.5 million), four reported collections of between one million and five million cards (greater than four million), and one reported a collection of six million for a conservative estimate of more than 13.5 million Guthrie cards stored in the United States, Puerto Rico, and the Virgin Islands. Tissues collected for diagnostic or therapeutic reasons may sometimes be used for research, educational, and quality-control purposes. However, the vast majority are not.

Several repositories have been established specifically for use in research (see "Large Banks, Repositories, and Core Facilities" in Appendixes A and C). In addition, several very large longitudinal studies collect and bank samples from their study participants. Likewise, a fair amount of research simultaneously creates tissue collections or contributes to tissue banks. Collectively, these contain more than 2.3 million specimens. Because these tissues are collected specifically for research purposes, it is not surprising that the use of these tissues has resulted in numerous research publications: more than 8,000 publications have resulted from the use of cells from the Coriell Institute; 2,000 publications have resulted from studies using tissues from the Cooperative Human Tissue Network (CHTN); and more than 632 publications, three textbooks, and numerous monographs have been produced using samples and data from the Bogalusa Heart Study.

Other than for diagnostic purposes or for use in research, tissues are also collected and stored for a variety of reasons. Blood banks collect approximately 12 million units of blood a year, but only about 20,000 to 40,000 units are stored at any one time. Also, most of the blood collected is used for transfusions. Very little is used for research and quality control. Organ banks do not collect the same volume of tissue that blood banks do but are very similar in the respect that most of the organs and tissues collected are used for transplants and very little is available for research. Forensic DNA banks collect and store tissues for use in criminal investigations. The DoD DNA Specimen Repository and some commercial DNA banks store DNA samples for remains identification. Sperm, ovum, and embryo banks store specimens for anonymous donation or for later use by the individual storing the material. Umbilical cord blood banks also store blood for anonymous donation and later use by families banking their newborns' cord blood.

Many valuable specimens and data resources exist from a variety of sources, but no centralized database allows researchers to obtain access to and information about them. The NCI is developing a national information database of breast cancer resources to centralize information on biological specimens available to the research and clinical community, promoting access to the specimens, and facilitating collaboration among basic, clinical, and epidemiologic researchers. This database will fulfill one of the priorities of the National Action Plan on Breast Cancer (NAPBC). However, this database is not an exhaustive national listing of all facilities holding breast cancer tissue but is limited to resources that have a breast tissue bank and have the capability and desire to provide tissues or to participate in collaborations.

This RAND national resource brings together information about several sources of stored tissue samples in the United States. It represents the first time that this information has been assembled in a single document and the first time the magnitude of the archives of stored tissues has been assessed. This document may serve as a reference for researchers to identify potential tissue resources. It may also serve as a basis for developing a national database.

QUANTITY OF STORED TISSUE SAMPLES IN THE UNITED STATES

Type of Repository/Institution	Number of Cases	Number of Specimens	Cases/Year
Large Tissue Banks, Repositories, and Core Facilities			
AFIP DNA Specimen Repository		>2.8 million	10,000
AFIP National Pathology Repository	>2.5 million	>92 million	50,000
Brain and Tissue Banks for Developmental Disorders	2,507	34,943	
Cancer Tissue Bank—VAMC Minneapolis		>2,000	
Case Western Reserve Alzheimer's Center		554	
Coriell Institute for Medical Research		>35,000	
Eastern Cooperative Oncology Group (ECOG)		18,000	3,000
Environmental Health Sciences Center	2,500	2,500	
Gastrointestinal SPORE—JHU		4,207	
Gynecologic Oncology Group Tissue Bank (GOG)	3,176	3,176	
Harvard Brain Tissue Resource Center/Harvard Psychiatry Brain Collection		>5,000	~350
HealthPartners Human Brain Bank	2,150	2,150	
Hereditary Disease Foundation	14,000	14,000	
Human Lung Cancer Tissue Resource		236	
Indiana Alzheimer Disease Center National Cell Repository	2,200	2,200	
Inflammatory Bowel Disease Tissue Bank	>250	>750	
Intergroup Rhabdomyosarcoma Study	>2,400	>2,400	
Kaiser Permanente Center for Health Research		>26,000	
Kathleen Price Bryan Brain Bank	900	900	
Kresge Center for Environmental Health Studies		53	
LifeSpan BioSciences, Inc.		1 million	
Lung Cancer in Uranium Miners: A Tissue Resource		248	
Lung Cancer SPORE—University of Colorado Cancer Center		>1,100	
McKesson BioServices		18.5 million	
Medical College of Georgia Human Brain Bank	24	912	5
Michigan's ADRC Brain Bank		300	50
National Human Monitoring Program	12,000	12,000	
National Neurological Research Specimen Bank	>11,000	>11,000	
National Psoriasis Tissue Bank		1,300	

Type of Repository/Institution	Number of Cases	Number of Specimens	Cases/Year
National Temporal Bone, Hearing, and Balance Pathology Resource Registry	>6,300	12,000	
National Wilms Tumor Study Group	440	440	
NCI AIDS Malignancy Bank	2,002	>18,000	
NCI Breast Cancer Specimen System	>130,000	>240,000	>460
NCI Cooperative Breast Cancer Tissue Resource	8,200	8,200	
NCI Cooperative Human Tissue Network (CHTN)		>100,000	
New York State Multiple Sclerosis Consortium		>1,000	
NHLBI Blood Specimen Repository		1.5 million	300,000
NIH AIDS Research and Reference Reagent Repository		17,000	
NIMH Brain Bank		1,200	
NIST Human Monitoring Program	12,000	12,000	
NIST National Biomonitoring Specimen Bank	661	661	
Oral Cancer Research Center—UCSF	>3,000	>3,000	125
PathServe Human Tissue Bank	300	30,000	300
Pediatric Oncology Group	>50,000	>50,000	
Prediagnostic Breast Cancer Serum Bank	>7,300	>7,300	
Program for Critical Technologies in Molecular Medicine		3 million	25,000
Prostate Cancer Tumor Bank		>1,030	
Radiation Therapy Oncology Group (RTOG)	(fixed) 4,400 (frozen) 70	4,700 290	1,500
Rocky Mountain Multiple Sclerosis Center Tissue Bank		170	
Rush Alzheimer's Disease Center		>1,000	
Southwest Oncology Group—Intergroup Breast Tissue Bank		>4,000	
St. Louis University Alzheimer's Brain Bank	1,000	1,000	
St. Luke's–Roosevelt Institute for Health Sciences	75	>75	
St. Paul–Ramsey Medical Center Brain Bank	>700	>700	
Stanley Foundation Brain Collection		>200	
Stanley Foundation Neuropathology Consortium		60	
State of Florida Brain Bank		>1,000	
Taub Center For Alzheimer's Disease Research Tissue Bank		300	
Texas Repository for AIDS Neuropathogenesis Research		450	
UCLA Alzheimer's Disease Center		>100	
UCSF AIDS Specimen Bank		76,000	
Western Genitourinary Tissue Bank		>250	
Wisconsin's Alzheimer's Disease Brain Tissue Bank		267	
Longitudinal Studies			
Bogalusa Heart Study	14,000	14,000	
Framingham Heart Study	5,209	5,209	
National Health and Nutrition Examination Surveys	85,000	85,000	
NIH Women's Health Initiative	168,000	>336,000	
The Nun Study	678	>678	
Physicians' Health Study	22,701	22,701	

Type of Repository/Institution	Number of Cases	Number of Specimens	Cases/Year
Women and Infants Transmission Study	2,200	>2,200	
Women's Health Study	40,000	40,000	
Women's Interagency HIV Study	2,300	>2,300	
Pathology Specimens			
Graduate Medical Education Teaching Institutions	>160 million	>160 million	>8 million
Newborn Screening Laboratories			
50 states, District of Columbia, Puerto Rico, and Virgin Islands	>13.5 million	>13.5 million	<10,000 to >500,000
Forensic DNA Banks			
48 states with Forensic DNA Banks	1.4 million	1.4 million	
Sperm, Ovum, and Embryo Banks			
California Cryobank	>200	>7,600	
Genetics and IVF Institute		2,300	2,300 embryos
Umbilical Cord Blood Banks			
American Cord Blood Program	>1,000	>1,000	
Chicago Community Cord Blood Bank	>300	>300	
Cord Blood Registry (CBR) & International Cord Blood Foundation (ICBF)	>8,000	>8,000	
New England Cord Blood Bank, Inc.	>200	>200	
New York Blood Center Placental Blood Program	7,000	7,000	
St. Louis Cord Blood Bank	>1,800	>1,800	
Organ Banks			
American Red Cross Tissue Services		>70,000	>70,000
Mid-America Transplant Services		>1,500	>1,500
Northwest Tissue Center		4,000	4,000
Blood Banks			
American Red Cross		~5.8 million	~5.8 million
Navy Blood Program		140,000	140,000
All Other Blood Banks		~6 million	~6 million

OVERALL SUMMARY OF STORED TISSUE SAMPLES
IN THE UNITED STATES

Type of Repository	Number of Cases	Number of Specimens	Cases/Year
Large Tissue Banks, Repositories, and Core Facilities	>2.8 million	>119.6 million	390,790
Longitudinal Studies	>340,088	>508,088	
Pathology Specimens	>160 million	>160 million	>8 million
Newborn Screening Laboratories	>13.5 million	>13.5 million	<10,000 to >50,000
Forensic DNA Banks	1.4 million	1.4 million	
Sperm, Ovum, and Embryo Banks	>>200	>9,900	>2,300
Umbilical Cord Blood Banks	>18,300	>18,300	
Organ Banks		>75,500	>75,500
Blood Banks		~12 million	~12 million
Grand Total	>178.0 million	>307.1 million	>20.5 million

SUMMARY OF TISSUE BANKS/REPOSITORIES
BY TISSUE TYPE

Table C.1

Summary of Tissue Banks/Repositories by Tissue Type

Tissue Group/ Resource	Number of Specimens/ Tissue Type(s)	Other Data	Limitations
Adipose			
National Human Adipose Tissue Survey	12,000 samples of adipose tissue from autopsied cadavers and surgical patients		
Brain			
Stanley Foundation Brain Collection	>200 brains from individuals with schizophrenia, bipolar disorders, severe depression, and normal controls Brains are half frozen, half formalin-fixed		
Stanley Foundation Neuropathology Consortium	60 brains: 15 each from individuals with schizophrenia, bipolar disorder, severe depression, and normal controls	Brains are distributed coded; on disclosure of results to consortium, codes will be supplied to researchers	
Harvard Brain Tissue Resource Center/Harvard Psychiatry Brain Collection—McLean Hospital	>5,000 brains from individuals mostly with Alzheimer's, Huntington's, or Parkinson's diseases Specimens are fresh quick-frozen tissue blocks and coronal sections, passive frozen hemispheres, or formalin-fixed hemispheres (researchers can request custom dissection of specified anatomic regions of passive frozen or formalin-fixed hemispheres	Age, gender, cause of death, postmortem time, and a neuropathology report (clinical records are available for approved investigators to read for themselves if they wish to visit the brain bank facility)	None specified

Table C.1— continued

Tissue Group/ Resource	Number of Specimens/ Tissue Type(s)	Other Data	Limitations
Alzheimer's Disease Research Center at Duke University— Kathleen Price Bryan Brain Bank	>600 brains from Alzheimer's patients or related causes of dementia >150 brains from patients with other neurological disorders (ALS, Huntington's, muscular dystrophy) 150 normal brains Fixed/frozen hemispheres, paraffin blocks, histological slides	Limited clinical information Demographic information	No distribution to third parties No cost except shipping fees
Taub Center for Alzheimer's Disease Research Tissue Bank	300 flash-frozen and fixed brain tissue specimens from patients with neurodegenerative disorders and normals Also store peripheral blood cells and DNA from patients with these disorders		
Boston University Alzheimer's Disease Center—Tissue Resource Center	Normal, demented, and diagnosed Alzheimer tissue samples available from frontal lobe, temporal lobe, parietal lobe, occipital lobe, motor lobe, somato-sensory lobe, visual lobe, olfactory cortex, insular cortex, spinal cord, cerebellum, putamen, prefrontal cortex, caudate, amygdala, hippocampus, and thalamus Specimens are flash-frozen or plp immersion fixed Brain endothelial cell cultures from rapid postmortem samples available	Extensive neurological data Demographic data	Specimens are for research purposes only; no portion of tissues may be given to third parties Any publication resulting from or related to use of tissues must acknowledge BU-ADC

Table C.1- continued

Tissue Group/ Resource	Number of Specimens/ Tissue Type(s)	Other Data	Limitations
Brain Bank—Medical College of Georgia	24 brains: 20 are Alzheimer's brains and the others are Parkinson's, other Lewy body disorders, and normals 1 hemisphere is sectioned and frozen, the other hemisphere has 18+ regions sampled with duplicative blocks fixed either in 10% NBF or 70% ETOH; some are paraffin-embedded Blood and DNA specimens from 138 individuals (48 Alzheimer's; 50 neurologic controls; the rest from different neurological disorders)	Some demographic data Clinical data on recently acquired cases	Does not provide tissues for commercial uses Shipping costs must be paid
HealthPartners Human Brain Bank	>2,000 frozen brain specimens from cases of Alzheimer's, Parkinson's, multi-infarction dementia, dementia with Lewy bodies, Pick's disease, unclassified dementia 150 normal controls	Sex, age, neuropathological diagnosis, and clinical diagnosis	No distribution to third parties or use in creating cell lines or commercial uses outside of center's research aims Collaboration usually required Other confidentiality restrictions and assurances that funds flow back into the research from any commercial collaborators Depends on circumstances—may be no cost to individuals, but pharmaceutical companies are required to pay collection, storage, and shipping costs
State of Florida Brain Bank	>1,000 brain specimens Fixed or frozen	Clinical data, age, sex, and race	Acknowledgment of tissue source Shipping costs must be paid
NIMH Brain Bank	450 specimens, mostly frozen; some are formalin-fixed, some are half frozen/half fixed	Demographic and clinical data	Protocol required; no commercial uses

Table C.1- continued

Tissue Group/ Resource	Number of Specimens/ Tissue Type(s)	Other Data	Limitations
Southern Illinois University School of Medicine's Center for Alzheimer's Disease Brain Bank	More than 400 brains, fixed and frozen (avg. 20 brains collected per year	Age, sex, clinical diagnosis	Collaboration required
Michigan Alzheimer's Disease Research Center Brain Bank	>300 frozen brains	Clinical and basic demographic data	Brain specimens are only available to qualified investigators
Blood			
POG—Acute Lymphoblastic Leukemia Cell Bank	Thousands of frozen cell suspensions from leukemia patients (avg. 500–600 cases per year)	Only information requested for project type will be disclosed if approved	Cells may only be used for proposed research project; no subsequent redistribution to other investigators or use for other projects allowed without obtaining permission Collaboration required Cost depends on what is requested
NHLBI Blood Specimen Repository	1.5 million well-characterized specimens of serum, plasma, and cells from NHLBI-sponsored studies	Basic study information	Can only use samples for specified research protocols; may not distribute samples to any other persons Investigator pays shipping costs Tissue source must be acknowledged
DoD DNA Specimen Repository for Remains Identification	2 million DNA specimens (2 bloodstain cards and 1 buccal swab for each individual)		

Table C.1- continued

Tissue Group/ Resource	Number of Specimens/ Tissue Type(s)	Other Data	Limitations
Breast			
NCI Cooperative Family Registry for Breast Cancer Studies (CFRBCS centers: Australian Breast Cancer Family Registry; New York Registry of Breast Cancer Families; Northern California Cooperative Family Registry; Ontario Registry for Studies of Familial Breast Cancer; Philadelphia Breast Cancer Registry; Utah Cooperative Breast Cancer Registry)	Paraffin-embedded breast and ovarian cancers, peripheral blood lymphocytes, serum, fresh-frozen tissue, and other biological fluids	Related family history (pedigrees)	CFRBCS repository and related databases are available for interdisciplinary and translational breast cancer research; material can only be used for approved protocol
	More than 5,600 families have been ascertained 2,458 affected specimens and 1,840 unaffected specimens available	Clinical, demographic, and epidemiological data	CFRBCS must be referenced in manuscript title
			Fees for processing, extracting, and shipping of specimens must be paid
NCI Cooperative Breast Cancer Tissue Resource (CBCTR) (CBCTR participating centers: Fox Chase Center, Philadelphia, Pennsylvania; Kaiser Research Foundation Institute, Portland, Oregon; University of Miami; Washington University, St. Louis, Missouri)	>8,200 cases of formalin-fixed, paraffin-embedded primary breast cancer tissues	Associated pathology and clinical data	Specimens may be used for research purposes only; tissues and their products cannot be sold for commercial purposes nor distributed to third parties for purposes of sale
	Cases represent all stages of disease from both sexes, all ages, and all races/ethnicities	Demographic data	Collaborations may be established between researchers and resource investigators to provide necessary additional services
		Outcome/follow-up data	$10/case plus a $2 to $10/slide charge plus shipping and handling fees

Table C.1- continued

Tissue Group/ Resource	Number of Specimens/ Tissue Type(s)	Other Data	Limitations
Breast Tissue Repository	21 breast tumor cell lines (18 derived from primary breast tissues; 3 from cultured metastatic breast tissues); 13 of the 21 tumor cell lines are paired cell lines with corresponding blood lymphocyte lines 25 primary cultures of normal epithelial and/or stromal mammary cells (5 correspond to tumor-derived cell lines)	Clinical and pathological features of breast tumors used for initiation of cell lines Extensive cellular, molecular, and genetic abnormalities data available Some pedigrees available	Tumor cell lines and lymphoblastoid cell lines available from ATCC; see ATCC limitations Costs are variable, see ATCC catalog
National Surgical Adjuvant Breast and Bowel Project (NSABP) Tissue Bank	Paraffin-embedded tumor specimens available from 25 NSABP trials; 40,479 cases enrolled: 18,529 with blocks or unstained slides; 36,242 with stained slides; and 17,240 with both	Complete clinical follow-up information as well as demographic information	Investigators with novel projects that conform to the research goals of NSABP may apply for tissue; priority given to NSABP membership institutions that regularly submit tissue blocks; tissue will not be distributed to commercial laboratories
Gastrointestinal			
Gastrointestinal Cancer at SPORE Johns Hopkins University	Banks wide range of tissue from resection specimens of colorectal and pancreatic cancer >716 colorectal cancer resections >142 colorectal adenoma resections >398 colorectal polypectomy specimens >47 hepatic resections for metastatic cancer >80 pancreatic cancer resections >107 fecal specimens >1,338 blood specimens	Family histories Food frequency data from questionnaire	

Table C.1- continued

Tissue Group/ Resource	Number of Specimens/ Tissue Type(s)	Other Data	Limitations
Inflammatory Bowel Disease Tissue Bank	>775 specimens from about 225 cases 150 cases are inflammatory bowel disease (Crohn's disease and ulcerative colitis); remainder are colon cancer, adeno-carcinoma, and diverticular disease	Final diagnosis Gross description of specimen Age and sex of patient	
Genital			
Gynecologic Tissue Group Tissue Bank	Benign, malignant, and normal ovarian and cervical tissue and serum from >3,176 patients Snap-frozen, formalin-fixed, OCT embedded primary tumors, touch imprint slides	Clinical Age, race Institutional pathology/ operative reports	
Hepatic			
NIST-EPA Human Liver Specimen Bank	661 normal liver specimens flash frozen	Demographic data Cause of death Histology report	Acknowledgment of tissue bank required Cost to be ascertained per proposal request
Liver Tissue Procurement and Distribution System	>1,500 frozen specimens from more than 60 types of diseased and normal livers	Demographic data Clinical data Family history (investigators should state areas of interest)	Samples are for NIH investigators only $110 per sample with each additional sample costing $15
Inclusive			
MGH Tumor Bank	>7,500 specimens have been collected and catalogued Normal and tumor specimens are snap-frozen	Verified pathologic diagnosis Some clinical information	$20/specimen

Table C.1- continued

Tissue Group/ Resource	Number of Specimens/ Tissue Type(s)	Other Data	Limitations
National Pathology Repository	50 million microscopic slides; 30 million paraffin tissue blocks; 12 million preserved wet tissue specimens Specimens represent the entire spectrum of human disease		Requests for loan of material or provision of data for research purposes require submission and approval of research protocol; request from individuals and organizations other than the original contributor must be accompanied by a properly executed authorization signed by the patient or designated representative
Yale Program for Critical Technologies in Molecular Medicine	More than 10,000 frozen tissue samples; more than 3 million archived paraffin blocks from clinical cases	Age, Sex, pathology diagnosis	Approved protocol by the Yale Human Investigation Committee; Material Transfer Agreement from non-Yale investigators; fee-for-service costs
NCI Cooperative Human Tissue Network (CHTN)	From 1987–1996, supplied >100,000 specimens to ~600 investigators Provides biomedical researchers access to fresh surgical or biopsy specimens of normal, benign, precancerous, and cancerous tissues; only rare specimens are stored to anticipated future requests	Minimal demographic information Histology/pathology reports	Tissues provided by the CHTN are only for research purposes and cannot be sold or used for commercial purposes
Radiation Therapy Oncology Group	Collects 3–5 frozen tissue fragments per case from Phase III protocols of cervical, lung, head and neck, esophageal, and anal cancers; >290 specimens from ~70 cases (two-thirds of specimens from cervical cancer) Beginning in 1995, RTOG archived paraffin blocks and tissues from all RTOG Phase III trials; tissue from ~4,400 cases have been collected and stored	No clinical information released that might allow for patient identification or linkage to treatment or demographics	Frozen tissue for use in correlative and translational research; paraffin blocks and tissues for population-based studies

Table C.1- continued

Tissue Group/ Resource	Number of Specimens/ Tissue Type(s)	Other Data	Limitations
NCI AIDS Malignancy Bank (research centers: Ohio State University, University of California—San Francisco, George Washington University, State University of New York, University of California—Los Angeles)	> 18,000 samples from >2,000 cases of HIV malignancy-related diseases Formalin-fixed paraffin-embedded tissues, fresh-frozen tissues, malignant cell suspensions, fine needle aspirate, cell lines Tissues include serum, plasma, urine, bone marrow, cervical and anal specimens, saliva, semen, and multisite autopsy tissues	Clinical data	Specimens may be used for research purposes only; specimens and their products shall not be sold or used for commercial purposes, nor be distributed to third parties for purposes of sale or producing for sale Shipping cost of specimens must be paid
Tumor Bank Facility at the Herbert Irving Comprehensive Cancer Center	Tumors and tumor/normal pairs Members can request specific types of tissue for their research protocols Tissues are snap frozen		Users must be Herbert Irving Comprehensive Cancer Center members
Brain and Tissue Bank for Developmental Disorders		Clinical data Demographic data	Tissue specimens may only be used for the specified study; research beyond that described in original request may only be carried out pursuant to another agreement signed by both parties; investigator shall not distribute tissue to third parties Acknowledgment of Brain and Tissue Bank for Developmental Disorders required Investigator will provide Director with written summary every 6 months on receipt of tissue Shipping and handling costs plus $50/ per tissue processing fees must be paid

Table C.1- continued

Tissue Group/ Resource	Number of Specimens/ Tissue Type(s)	Other Data	Limitations
University of Maryland, Baltimore	12,000 brain sections; 53 body fluids; 1,500 cardiovascular tissue; 1,300 endocrine tissue; 6,000 gastrointestinal tissue; 700 genital tissue; 1,600 hematopoietic tissue; 1,000 integumentary tissue; 1,800 musculoskeletal tissue; 2,000 respiratory tissue; 1,900 spinal cord tissue; 1,600 urinary tissue; 800 other types of tissue		
	Tissue samples are frozen or fixed		
University of Miami	All tissue types from 854 cases of 142 disease types and normals		
	Myoblast, fibroblast and/or lymphoblast cell cultures exist from some cases		
Children's Hospital of Orange County	Currently have tissues and/or cultured cells from >800 patients of 253 disease types and normals		
DAIDS Specimen Repository			Collaboration required
Multicenter AIDS Cohort Study	Cells, serum, plasma, tissue (lymph node biopsies and autopsy tissues), semen, throat washings, fecal scrubs		
Women and Infants Transmission Study	Adult specimens include blood, urine, genital samples, Pediatric specimens include blood and urine		
Women's Interagency Health Study	Blood, oral/pharyngeal swabs, urine, vaginal and cervical swabs, cervicovaginal lavage fluids		

Table C.1- continued

Tissue Group/ Resource	Number of Specimens/ Tissue Type(s)	Other Data	Limitations
HIV Network for Prevention Trials	Serum, plasma, peripheral mononuclear cells, genital tract secretions, saliva (HIV strains isolated from these tissues also available)		
Pediatric AIDS Clinical Trials Group	Serum, plasma, peripheral mononuclear cells, culture supernatants, lymph node biopsies, tissues, urine, and other body fluids		
Adult AIDS Clinical Trials Group	Serum, plasma, peripheral blood mononuclear cells, culture supernatants, lymph node biopsies, tissues, urine, and other body fluids		
AIDS Vaccine Evaluation Group	Serum, plasma, peripheral mononuclear cells, genital tract secretions, saliva, and tears		
Division of AIDS Treatment Research Initiative	Serum, plasma, cells and cultured cells, supernatant from PBMC, plasma HIV cultures		
National Neurological Research Specimen Bank	Tissue specimens and CSF and blood collected from more than 11,000 cases Includes brain, spinal cord, pituitary glands, thymus, spleen, eyes, and lymph nodes	Confirmed diagnosis Demographic data	Tissue specimens distributed to approved investigators only Acknowledgment of the bank is required Shipping costs must be paid
UCSF AIDS Specimen Bank	>76,000 specimens Serum, tissue, saliva, CSF from HIV-infected individuals		

Table C.1- continued

Tissue Group/ Resource	Number of Specimens/ Tissue Type(s)	Other Data	Limitations
Tissue Procurement Shared Resource at Ohio State University Comprehensive Cancer Center (CCC)	Handled >75,000 specimens (avg. 3,000/yr) Investigators can request remnant surgical or autopsy tissue by filling out request form	Pathology report	Application approval requires approved human subjects IRB Costs for CCC full members— $5/specimen, CCC associate members—$8/specimen, CCC non-members—$10/specimen Single chart review—$25 Histology Q.C.—$7.85/tissue
LifeSpan BioSciences, Inc.— Tissue and Disease Bank	1,000,000 normal and diseased human samples >175 different types of tissue from almost every organ, covering all ages >1,500 different pathologic disease categories	Pathologic report and result from requested test	LifeSpan does not sell its tissue per se but performs custom services using its tissue bank Cost varies according to services requested
PathServe—Autopsy and Tissue Bank	Collects all types of organs and tissues including specimens from placental and fetal origin Has ~300 specimens stored at any one time (does not maintain a central storage facility but instead stores samples in morgues in different hospitals) distributed ~30,000 specimens last year	Limited medical history	Tissue may be unsuitable for RNA isolation due to degradation Recipient will use tissue for scientific/medical research only No distribution of tissues to third parties Costs are adult brain—$320, adult brain (cut)—$90, spinal cord—$240, heart—$320, tissue section (internal organs)—$240, artery—$59, placenta—$89, fetus—$290, fetal brain—$250, skin—$270, pericardium—$270, dura matter—$79, eyes (pair)—$240, temporal bones—$100, formalin-fixed block—$97

Table C.1- continued

Tissue Group/Resource	Number of Specimens/Tissue Type(s)	Other Data	Limitations
Resource for Tumor Tissue and Data—NYU Medical Center	Tissue specimens are collected per investigator needs (tumor specimens may be stored and frozen if no immediate need exists) Specimens can be snap-frozen or fixed; tissue paraffin blocks also available	Specific clinical and/or demographic data are made available Pathology reports	Unused sections of paraffin blocks must be returned upon completion of the study
Musculoskeletal			
National Temporal Bone, Hearing and Balance Pathology Resource Registry	>12,000 temporal bone and brain tissue specimens from more than 6,300 cases of hearing and balance disorders	Demographic data Processing data Clinical and histopathological diagnosis	Only the 26 collaborating temporal bone laboratories have access to bone specimens Researchers wishing to use bone specimens must contact the lab director and discuss their intentions
Baylor College of Medicine	1,040 temporal bones from 1,040 cases		
Bowman-Gray School of Medicine	1,074 temporal bones from 1,075 cases		
The Eye & Ear Institute of Pittsburgh	1,385 temporal bones from 826 cases		
Goodhill Ear Center at UCLA School of Medicine	1,000 temporal bones from 500 cases; 10 brain specimens		
House Ear Institute	1,256 temporal bones from 2,008 cases; 72 brain specimens		
Kresge Hearing Research Institute-University of Michigan	60 temporal bones from 65 cases; 4 brain specimens		
Johns Hopkins University	3,520 temporal bones from 3,522 cases; 2 brain specimens		

Table C.1-   continued

Tissue Group/ Resource	Number of Specimens/ Tissue Type(s)	Other Data	Limitations
Massachusetts Eye and Ear Infirmary	1,518 temporal bones from 862 cases		
Mount Sinai School of Medicine	Not reported		
New York University	300 temporal bones from 300 cases		
SUNY Health Science Center-Syracuse	198 temporal bones from 162 cases		
University of Chicago	1,600 temporal bones from 771 cases: 293 brain specimens		
University of Iowa Hospitals and Clinics	818 temporal bones from 818 cases		
University of Minnesota	1,694 temporal bones from 946 cases		
University of Texas South-western Medical Center	Temporal bones from 137 cases		
Other Biological Materials (Cells, DNA, RNA, protein)			
NIH AIDS Research and Reference Reagent Program (AIDS Reagent Program)	>1,400 reagents available, including HIV and related viruses, opportunistic infectious agents associated with HIV infections, DNA libraries, DNA clones, antibodies, purified proteins, synthetic peptides, and body fluids		Any commercial use requires written permission and compensation of reagent donor(s) and notification of the AIDS Reagent Program; investigators must register with NIH AIDS Research and Reference Reagent Program Investigator pays shipping costs

Table C.1- continued

Tissue Group/ Resource	Number of Specimens/ Tissue Type(s)	Other Data	Limitations
Indiana Alzheimer Disease Center National Cell Repository	Genetic material from more than 2,200 individuals from 440 families with histories of Alzheimer's disease (both lymphocytes and DNA are available from most participants)	Family pedigrees	Asked to cite IADC National Cell Repository Researchers may not transfer cells or DNA to third parties Materials received from IADC National Cell Repository may not be used for commercial purposes
Human Genetic Mutant Cell Repository (Coriell Cell Repositories)	Contains both DNA and cells from human and animal cultures, normal controls, inherited disorders and normal variants, NIGMS extended family collections		Recipient agrees not to try to identify or contact submitter of sample or the donor subject from whom the cell line or DNA is derived; products derived from human cell cultures and DNA samples from HGMCR may not be sold or distributed with or without charge to third party Acknowledgment of repository in publications is required Costs are cell cultures—$75, human DNA—$50, hybrid DNA—$150

Table C.1- continued

Tissue Group/Resource	Number of Specimens/Tissue Type(s)	Other Data	Limitations
NIA Cell Repository (Coriell Cell Repositories)	Cell cultures from aging syndromes, Alzheimer's, normals, fibroblasts from aged sibling pairs, other cell types, animal cells	Each shipment includes a computer generated information sheet describing cell culture	Recipient agrees to obtain written permission of submitter and U.S. government before commercialization of cell lines or any products; cell cultures obtained cannot be resold, or distributed free of charge, but they may be replicated by a third party for the original purchaser Costs are T25 flask—$75 (for larger orders, first 75 are $75 and each additional culture is $25)
ADA Cell Repository Maturity Onset Diabetes Collection	DNA samples and phenotypic data from Phase I and II of the ADA's GENNID study—data on 170 pedigrees with a total of 650 affected individuals and approximately 1,200 subjects	Data set includes multiple metabolic factors as well as lifestyle variables	
American Tissue Culture Collection	Cell cultures from human, animal, and hybridomas	Basic description of cell culture (where derived, genotype, growth conditions)	Cost depends on type of cell culture ($50–$150) plus shipping and handling

ALPHABETICAL LISTING OF TISSUE BANKS/REPOSITORIES
AND CONTACTS

Tissue Bank	Address and Web Site
Albert Einstein College of Medicine Dept. of Pathology and Neuroscience	1300 Morris Park Ave. Bronx, NY 10461 Phone: 212-430-2827
Alpers Neuropathology Laboratory	Dept. of Neurology Thomas Jefferson University 130 S. 9th St., Suite 400 Philadelphia, PA 19107 Phone: 215-955-6939
Alzheimer's Center—Case Western Reserve University	11100 Euclid Ave. Cleveland, OH 44106 Phone: 216-844-7360 Fax: 216-844-7239 http://www.ohioalzcenter.org
Alzheimer Disease Center—Indiana University	Indiana University School of Medicine 635 Barnhill Dr., MS-A142 Indianapolis, IN 46202 Phone: 317-274-7818 Fax: 317-274-4882 Indiana Alzheimer Disease Center National Cell Repository Fax: 317-274-2387 http://medgen.iupui.edu/research/alzheimer
Alzheimer's Disease Center—University of California, Los Angeles	Dept. of Neurology 710 Westwood Plaza Los Angeles, CA 90095 Phone: 310-206-5238 Fax: 310-206-5287
Alzheimer's Disease Center—Northwestern University	Northwestern University Medical School 320 E. Superior St. Searle 11-453 Chicago, IL 60611 Phone: 312-908-8789 Fax: 312-908-8789 http://www.brain.nwu.edu/core/index.htm

Tissue Bank	Address and Web Site
Alzheimer's Disease Center—University of Rochester	Dept. of Neurobiology & Anatomy Box 603 601 Elmwood Ave. Rochester, NY 14642 Phone: 716-275-2581 Fax: 716-273-1132
Alzheimer's Disease Center—University of Kansas Medical Center	Dept. of Neurology 3901 Rainbow Blvd. Kansas City, Kansas 66160 Phone: 913-588-6970 Fax: 913-588-6965 http://www.kumc.edu/instruction/medicine/ neurology/resAD.html
Alzheimer's Disease Center—University of California, Davis	Northern California Alzheimer's Disease Center Alta Bates Medical Center 2001 Dwight Way Berkeley, CA 94704 Phone: 510-204-4530 Fax: 510-204-4524 http://alzheimer.ucdavis.edu/adc
Alzheimer's Disease Core Center—Boston University	Geriatric, Education, and Clinical Center Bedford VA Medical Center 200 Springs Rd. Bedford, MA 01730 Phone: 781-687-2959 Fax: 781-687-3527 http://www.visn1.org/alzheimer/BrainBank.htm
Alzheimer's Disease Research Center—Baylor College of Medicine	ADRC 6560 Fannin St. Smith Tower, #1801 Houston, TX 77030 Phone: 713-798-6660 Fax: 713-798-5326 http://www.bcm.tmc.edu/neurol.struct/adrc/ adrc1.html
Alzheimer's Disease Research Center—University of Southern California	2011 Zonal Ave. Los Angeles, CA 90033 Phone: 310-442-1601 Fax: 323-442-1808 http://www.usc.edu/dept/gero/ARDC
Alzheimer's Disease Research Center—Washington University	Campus Box 8111—ADRC 660 South Euclid Ave. St. Louis, MO 63110 Phone: 314-362-2881 Fax: 314-362-4763 http://www.adrc.wustl.edu/adrc/adrc2.html

Tissue Bank	Address and Web Site
Alzheimer's Disease Research Center—University of Washington	Dept. of Pathology Box 357470 Seattle, WA 98195 Phone: 206-543-5088 Fax: 206-685-8356
Alzheimer's Tissue Repository I.R.U. in Brain Aging	University of California, Irvine Dept. of Psychobiology Irvine, CA 92717 Phone: 714-856-5032
Alzheimer's Treatment & Research Center	St. Paul–Ramsey Medical Ctr. 640 Jackson St. St. Paul, MN 48104-1687 Phone: 612-221-2743
Armed Forces Institute of Pathology	AFIP, Bldg. 54 Washington, D.C. 20306-6000 http://www.afip.org/
Armed Forces DNA Laboratory	[Armed Forces DNA Laboratory—http://www.afip.org/homes/oafme/dna/afdil.html]
National Pathology Repository	[National Pathology Repository—http://www.afip.org/Consultation/Standard_Consultation/Repository_and_Research_Servic/national_pathology_repository_.html]
Biologic Specimen Bank	Research Institute on Addictions 1021 Main St. Buffalo, NY 14203
Brain and Tissue Bank for Developmental Disorders—Children's Hospital of Orange County	455 South Main St. Orange, CA 92868 Phone: 1-800-992-2462 Fax. 714-532-8442 http://www.choc.com/btbmain.htm
Brain and Tissue Bank for Developmental Disorders—University of Maryland	Bressler Research Building #10-35 655 W. Baltimore St. Baltimore, MD 21201 Phone: 800-847-1539 Fax: 410-706-0020 http://www.som1.umaryland.edu/BTBank
Brain and Tissue Bank for Developmental Disorders—University of Miami	Dept. of Pathology, 410 Pap Bldg. (R-5) 1550 N.W. 10th Ave. Miami, FL 33136 Phone: 800-592-7246 Fax: 305-243-6970 http://www.med.miami.edu/BTB

Tissue Bank	Address and Web Site
Brain Bank—Medical College of Georgia	Medical College of Georgia Augusta, GA 30912 Phone: 706-721-2019 Fax: 706-721-6839 http://www.mcg.edu/Centers/Alz/arc.htm
Brain Tumor and Tissue Bank—University of Cincinnati College of Medicine; Dept. of Pathology and Laboratory Medicine	231 Bethesda Ave. Cincinnati, OH 45267-0524 Phone: 513-558-7109
CALGB Leukemia Tissue Bank	The Arthur G. James Cancer Hospital & Research Institute 320 West 10th Ave. Room 458A, Starling-Loving Hall Columbus, OH 43210 Phone: 614-293-7521 Fax: 614-293-7522 [Central Office—http://128.135.31.4]
California NeuroAIDS Tissue Network	University of California, San Diego Stein Research Bldg. 9500 Gilman Dr. San Diego, CA 92093
Center for Alzheimer's Disease and Related Disorders	PO Box 19230 Southern Illinois School of Medicine Springfield, IL 62794-9230 Phone: 217-524-6719
Center for Neurological Diseases	Brigham & Women's Hospital 75 Francis St. Boston, MA 02115 Phone: 617-732-6454
ECOG Solid Tumor Tissue Bank/Leukemia Tissue Bank	ECOG Coordinating Center FSTRF 303 Boylston St. Brookline, MA 02445 Phone: 617-632-3610 Fax: 617-632-2990
Emory University's Alzheimer's Disease Center	VA Medical Center 1670 Clairmont Rd. Decatur, GA 30033 Phone: 404-728-7714 Fax: 404-728-7771 http://www.emory.edu/WHSC/MED/ADC
Geriatric Neurobehavior and Alzheimer's Center	University of Southern California 12838 Erickson Ave. Downey, CA 90342 Phone: 310-940-7094 Fax: 310-803-0921

Tissue Bank	Address and Web Site
GOG Tissue Bank	Children's Hospital Research Foundation 700 Children's Dr. Columbus, OH 43205 Phone: 614-722-5302 Fax: 614-722-2897 http://www.gog.org
GOG/CHTN Ovarian Tissue Bank	Children's Hospital, J058 700 Children's Dr. Columbus, OH 43205 Phone: 614-722-2890 Fax: 614-722-2897 http://www.gog.org
Harvard Brain Tissue Resource Center	McLean Hospital 115 Mill St. Belmont, MA 02178 Phone: 617-855-2400 http://www.mcleanhospital.org/ brainbank.html
HealthPartners Human Brain Bank	Alzheimer's Research Center Regions Hospital Foundation 640 Jackson St. St. Paul, MN 55101 Phone: 800-229-2872 Fax: 651-292-4040
Indiana University Medical Center Division of Neuropathology	635 Barnhill Dr., MS A142 Indianapolis, IN 46233 Phone: 317-274-7818
Inflammatory Bowel Disease Tissue Bank	Massachusetts General Hospital 55 Fruit St., Warren 256 Boston, MA 02114 Phone: 617-724-0277
Institute of Pathology	Case Western Reserve University 2085 Adelbert Rd. Cleveland, OH 44106 Phone: 216-844-1808
Kathleen Price Bryan Brain Bank	Dept. of Pathology, Box 3712 Duke University Medical Ctr. Durham, NC 27710 Phone: 919-684-5963 [Located within Duke's ADRC— http://www.medicine.mc.duke.edu/ADRC/ INDEX.html]
LifeSpan BioSciences, Inc.	700 Blanchard St. Seattle, WA 98121 Phone: 206-464-1554 Fax: 206-464-1723 http://www.lsbio.com

Tissue Bank	Address and Web Site
LSU Neuroscience Center Brain Tissue Bank	2020 Gravier LSU Medical Center New Orleans, LA 70112 Phone: 504-599-0916 http://neuroscience.lsumc.edu/BrainBank.html
Manhattan HIV Brain Bank	Mt. Sinai School of Medicine New York, New York 10029
Massachusetts General Hospital Dept. of Neurology	Massachusetts General Hospital Dept. of Neurology, Warren 321 55 Fruit St. Boston, MA 02114 Phone: 617-726-5154
Massachusetts General Hospital Tumor Bank	Division of Hematology/Oncology Jackson 1021 MGH 55 Fruit St. Boston, MA 02114 Phone: 617-724-7081 Fax: 617-726-6974 http://cancer.mgh.harvard.edu/tumorbank
Mayo Clinic Dept. of Pathology	200 First St., S.W. Rochester, MN 55905 Phone: 507-284-6828
Mayo Clinic Jacksonville	4500 San Pablo Rd. Jacksonville, FL 32224 Phone: 904-223-2000
Michigan Alzheimer's Disease Research Center	Dept. of Neurology Michigan Alzheimer's Disease Research Ctr. University of Michigan 1103 E. Huron St. Ann Arbor, MI 48104-1687 Phone: 734-764-5479 Fax: 734-764-2189 http://www.med.umich.edu/madrc/ MADRC.html
Missouri Lions Eye Research Foundation	404 Portland St. Columbia, MO 65201 Phone: 573-443-1471 www.rollanet.org/~rlions/mlerf
Mt. Sinai School of Medicine Dept. of Psychiatry	One Gustave L. Levy Pl. New York, NY 10029-6571 Phone: 212-584-9000, ext. 1789

Tissue Bank	Address and Web Site
Mucosal Immunology Core	11-934 Factor Building Box 951678 Los Angeles, CA 90095 Phone: 310-206-5797 Fax: 310-206-8824 http://www.medsch.ucla.edu/aidsinst/cfar/ Mucosal.htm
National Disease Research Interchange— Human Tissues and Organs for Research; Human Biological Data Interchange; Odyssey One	2401 Walnut St. Suite 408 Philadelphia, PA 19103 Phone: 800-222-NDRI http://www.ndri.com
National Neurological AIDS Bank	W127 Neurology VAMC Los Angeles, CA 90073
National Neurological Research Bank	VA Wadsworth Medical Ctr. Wilshire and Sawtelle Blvds. Los Angeles, CA 90073 Phone: 213-824-4307
National Neurological Research Specimen Bank	VA Greater Los Angeles HealthCare System West Los Angeles VA Medical Center 11301 Wilshire Blvd. Los Angeles, CA 90073 Phone: 310-268-3536 Fax: 310-268-4768 http://www.loni.ucla.edu/~nnrsb/nnrsb
National Psoriasis Tissue Bank	Phone: 800-723-9166 ext. 13 Fax: 503-245-0626 http://www.psoriasis.org/tissuebank.html
National Surgical Adjuvant Breast and Bowel Project (NSABP)	NSABP Operations Center East Commons Professional Bldg. Four Allegheny Center—5th Floor Pittsburgh, PA 15212 Phone: 412-330-4600 Fax: 412-330-4660 http://www.nsabp.pitt.edu/
National Wilms Tumor Study Group Tissue Bank	Dept. of Pediatrics Roswell Park Cancer Institute Elm and Carlton Sts. Buffalo, NY 14263 Phone: 716-845-2334 Fax: 716-845-8003
Neuropathology Autopsy Core	University of Southern California 2011 Zonal Ave. Los Angeles, CA 90033 Phone: 213-342-1602

Tissue Bank	Address and Web Site
New York University Medical Center Dept. of Pathology	550 First Ave. New York, NY 10016 Phone: 212-263-6449
Ohio St. University College of Medicine Division of Neuropathology	N-112B Upham Hall 473 W. 12th Ave. Columbus, OH 43210 Phone: 614-293-8254
Oregon Health Sciences University Division of Neuropathology	3181 S.W. Sam Jackson Park Rd., L113 Portland, OR 97201 Phone: 503-494-4654
PathServe Autopsy & Tissue Bank	PO Box 22023 San Francisco, CA 94122 Phone: 415-664-9686 Fax: 415-664-5861 http://www.tissuebank.com
POG ALL Cell Bank	Stanford University School of Medicine Mail Code 5208 300 Pasteur Dr. Stanford, CA 94305 Phone: 650-723-5535 Fax: 650-498-6937
POG AML Cell Bank	St. Jude Children's Research Hospital 332 N. Lauderdale St. Memphis, TN 38105 Phone: 901-495-2799 Fax: 901-495-3100
POG CNS Tumor Bank	Duke University Pediatric Neuro-Oncology Division Box 3624 Duke South Hospital Room 2228 Durham, NC 27710 Phone: 919-684-5301 Fax: 919-684-6674
POG Germ Cell Tumor Bank	University of Alabama Pediatric/Hem/Onc 1600 7th Ave. S. Suite 651 Birmingham, AL 35266 Phone: 205-939-9285 Fax: 205-975-6377
POG Hepatoblastoma Biology Study and Tissue Bank	University of Texas Southwestern Medical Center 5323 Harry Hines Blvd. Dallas, TX 75235 Phone: 214-648-4907 Fax: 214-648-4940

Tissue Bank	Address and Web Site
POG Hodgkin's Disease Bank	Wake Forest University School of Medicine Department of Pediatrics Medical Center Boulevard Winston-Salem, NC 27157 Phone: 336-716-4085 Fax: 336-716-3010
POG Lymphoid Relapse Cell Bank	MCSD Medical Center 200 W. Arbor Dr. San Diego, CA 92130 Phone: 619-543-6844 Fax: 619-543-5413
POG Neuroblastoma Bank	Division of Hematology/Oncology Box #30 Children's Memorial Hospital 2300 Children's Plaza Chicago, IL 60614 Phone: 773-880-4562 Fax: 773-880-3053
POG NHL Cell Bank	University of Massachusetts Medical School Pediatrics 55 Lake Ave. N. Worcester, MA 01655 Phone: 508-856-4225 Fax: 508-856-4282
POG Operations Office	645 N. Michigan Ave. Suite 910 Chicago, IL 60611 Phone: 312-482-9944 Fax: 312-482-9460 http://www.pog.ufl.edu
Resource for Tumor Tissue and Data NYU School of Medicine	Kaplan Comprehensive Cancer Center 550 First Ave. New York, NY 10016 Phone: 212-263-6452 Fax: 212-263-7573 http://kccc-www.med.nyu.edu/RTTD.htm
RTOG Tissue Bank	LDS Hospital 8th Ave. and C St. Salt Lake City, UT 84143 Phone: 801-321-1929 Fax: 617-632-5710
Rush Alzheimer's Disease Center (Rush Brain Bank)	Rush-Presbyterian–St. Luke's Medical Center 1653 W. Congress Pkwy. Chicago, IL 60612 Phone: 312-942-3350 http://www.rush.edu/Departments/ Alzheimers/Research.html

Tissue Bank	Address and Web Site
Rush Presbyterian St. Luke's Medical Center Dept. of Pathology	1653 W. Congress Pkwy. Chicago, IL 60612-3864 Phone: 312-942-5254
S.L.U.M.C./Alzheimer's Association Brain Bank	Dept. of Psychiatry and Human Behavior St. Louis University Medical Ctr. 1221 S. Grand Blvd. St. Louis, MO 63104 Phone: 314-577-8726
Sanders-Brown Research Center on Aging University of Kentucky	101 Sanders-Brown Bldg. Lexington, KY 40536 Phone: 606-223-6040
St. Louis University Alzheimer's Brain Bank	Dept. of Geriatric Psychiatry Wohl Memorial Institute 2nd Floor 1221 South Grand Blvd. St. Louis, MO 63104 Phone: 314-577-8719
State of Florida Brain Bank	Mt. Sinai Medical Center 4300 Alton Rd. Miami Beach, FL 33140 Phone: 305-674-2543
Sun Health Research Institute —Institute for Biogerontological Research	PO Box 1278 Sun City, AZ 85372 Phone: 602-876-5328 Fax: 602-876-5461
SWOG National Tissue Repository	Operations Office Southwest Oncology Group 14980 Omicron Dr. San Antonio, TX 78245 Phone: 210-677-8808 Fax: 210-677-0006
Taub Center for Alzheimer's Disease Research—Columbia University	Columbia-Presbyterian Medical Center 630 W. 168th St. New York, NY 10032 Phone: 212-305-4531 Fax: 212-305-4548 http://pathology.cpmc.columbia.edu/ ADNP.html
Texas Repository for AIDS Neuropathogenesis Research	University of Texas Medical Branch, Galveston 301 University Blvd. Galveston, TX 77550
Tissue Accrual and In Situ Imaging Core	The Wistar Institute 3601 Spruce St. Philadelphia, PA 19104
Tissue Culture Core	Weill Medical College of Cornell University New York, New York 10021

Tissue Bank	Address and Web Site
Tissue Procurement Core Facility	Dartmouth College Hanover, NH 03755
Tissue Procurement, Products, Bank, and Database—Yale University School of Medicine	
UCSD National Alzheimer's Disease Brain Bank	Dept. Pathology, M-012 BSB, Room 1004 University of California San Diego La Jolla, CA 92093 Phone: 619-534-6858 Fax: 619-534-8852
UCSF Cancer Center Tissue Core	Tissue Core UCSF Cancer Center Box 0808 San Francisco, CA 94143 Phone: 415-476-0435 http://cc.ucsf.edu/tissue/index.html
U.K.K.C. Neurodegeneration Autopsy Program	Dept. of Pathology U.K.K.C. Neurodegeneration Autopsy Program Truman Medical Ctr. 2301 Holmes St. Kansas City, MO 64108 Phone: 816-556-3212
University of California San Diego Dept. of Neuroscience and Pathology	UCSD 9500 Gilman Dr., Med. Tech. Bldg. 350 La Jolla, CA 92093 Phone: 619-534-6208 Fax: 619-534-6232
University of Florida Dept. of Neurology	1501 N.W. Ninth Ave. Miami, FL 33101 Phone: 305-547-6219
University of Iowa College of Medicine Dept. of Anatomy	650 Newton Rd. Iowa City, IA 52242 Phone: 319-335-7741
University of Massachusetts Dept. of Neurology	55 Lave Ave., North Worcester, MA 01655 Phone: 508-856-3323
University of Tennessee Medical Ctr.	1924 Alcoa Highway Knoxville, TN 37920 Phone: 615-544-9349
University of Texas at El Paso	206 Psychology Bldg. El Paso, TX 79968 Phone: 915-747-5551
University of Texas Southwestern Medical Ctr. Dept. of Pathology—Neuropathology Laboratory	5323 Harry Hines Blvd. Dallas, TX 75235-9072 Phone: 214-688-2148

Tissue Bank	Address and Web Site
University of Washington Dept. of Pathology	Dept. of Pathology, SM-30 Seattle, WA 98195 Phone: 206-543-1871
Washington Univ. School of Medicine Dept. of Pathology, Autopsy Service	Dept. of Pathology, Box 8118 Washington Univ. School of Medicine 660 S. Euclid Ave. St. Louis, MO 63110 Phone: 314-362-7440 Fax: 314-362-4096
Western Psychiatric Institute and Clinic	3811 O'Hara St., Room E-1230 Pittsburgh, PA 15213 Phone: 412-624-5186
Wisconsin Alzheimer's Disease Brain Tissue Bank	Medical College of Wisconsin 9200 W. Wisconsin Ave. Milwaukee, WI 53226 Phone: 414-454-5200 Fax: 414-259-0469
Zablocki V.A. Medical Center	Research Service 151 Milwaukee, WI 53295 Phone: 414-259-2881

ALPHABETICAL LISTING BY STATE OF TISSUE BANKS
DESCRIBED IN CHAPTER THREE

Alabama	Birmingham VA Medical Center—Early Detection Research Network: Tissue Bank for Matched Tissues to Screen for Markers of Neoplastic Progression
California	The International Skeletal Dysplasia Registry
	NCI AIDS Malignancy Bank
	UCLA Alzheimer's Disease Center
	University of Southern California—Environmental Health Sciences Center
	University of California, Davis—Institute of Toxicology and Environmental Health
	University of California, San Francisco—AIDS Specimen Bank
	Gift of Hope Brain Bank for AIDS
	Mucosal Immunology Core—UCLA
	Children's Hospital of Orange County—Brain and Tissue Bank for Developmental Disorders
	UCSF—Oral Cancer Research Center
	UCSF Cancer Center Tissue Core
	UCLA—Breast Tumor Bank
	Clontech
	Hereditary Disease Foundation
	National Neurological Research Specimen Bank
	PathServe Autopsy & Tissue Bank
Colorado	University of Colorado Cancer Center—SPORE in Lung Cancer
	Rocky Mountain Multiple Sclerosis Center Tissue Bank
Connecticut	Yale University—Program for Critical Technologies in Breast Oncology
District of Columbia	Armed Forces Institute of Pathology
	Georgetown University Medical Center and Lombardi Cancer Center—Breast Cancer Specimen Bank
	George Washington University—HIV-Related Malignancy Tissue/Biological Fluids Bank
	The Stanley Brain Collection and Neuropathology Consortium
Florida	University of Miami—Brain and Tissue Bank for Developmental Disorders
	State of Florida Brain Bank

Georgia	Emory University's Alzheimer's Disease Center
	Medical College of Georgia—Alzheimer's Research Center Brain Bank
Illinois	ECOG Solid Tumor Tissue Bank
Iowa	Iowa City VA Medical Center—Mental Health Clinic Research Center Brain Bank
Kansas	The University of Kansas Medical Center Alzheimer's Disease Center
Kentucky	Lexington VA Medical Center—Central Prostate Cancer Serum Repository
Louisiana	LSU's Stanley S. Scott Cancer Center—Tumor Bank for Solid Tumors
	LSU Neuroscience Center Brain Tissue Bank
Maryland	American Type Tissue Culture Collection
	Biomedical Research Institute
	Johns Hopkins University—SPORE in Gastrointestinal Cancer
	Johns Hopkins University—SPORE in Prostate Cancer
	Maryland Brain Collection
	McKesson BioServices
	National Biomonitoring Specimen Bank
	National Human Adipose Tissue Survey
	NCI Cooperative Breast Cancer Tissue Resource (CBCTR)
	NCI Prediagnostic Breast Cancer Serum Bank
	NCI Surveillance, Epidemiology, and End Results Program (SEER)
	NCI—Cooperative Central Nervous System Consortium Tissue Bank
	NCI—Biologic Specimen Bank for Early Lung Cancer Markers in Chinese Tin Miners
	NHLBI Blood Specimen Repository
	NIH National AIDS Research and Reference Reagent Program
	NIMH Brain Bank
	University of Maryland—Brain and Tissue Bank for Developmental Disorders
Massachusetts	Boston University's Alzheimer's Disease Center
	Dana Farber Cancer Institute — Breast Cancer Specimen Bank
	Harvard Brain Tissue Resource Center
	Harvard University—Kresge Center for Environmental Health Studies
	Inflammatory Bowel Disease Tissue Bank
	Massachusetts Eye and Ear Infirmary—National Temporal Bone, Hearing and Balance Pathology Resource Registry
	Massachusetts General Hospital Tumor Bank
Michigan	Michigan's Alzheimer's Disease Research Center Brain Bank
	University of Michigan Comprehensive Cancer Center—SPORE in Prostate Cancer
	University of Michigan—Breast Cell/Tissue Bank Data and Database
	University of Michigan—Tissue Procurement Core
	University of Michigan—Tissue/Pathology Core
Minnesota	North Central Cancer Treatment Group—Breast Cancer Specimen Bank
	HealthPartners Human Brain Bank
	Minneapolis VA Medical Center—Cancer Tissue Bank

Missouri	Washington University Alzheimer Disease Research Center
Nebraska	University of Nebraska Medical Center—SPORE in Gastrointestinal Cancer
New Hampshire	Dartmouth College—Tissue Procurement Core Facility
New Jersey	Coriell Institute for Medical Research
New Mexico	Albuquerque VA Medical Center—Human Lung Cancer Tissue Resource
	Albuquerque VA Medical Center—Lung Cancer in Uranium Miners: A Tissue Resource
New York	Kaplan Comprehensive Cancer Center at NYU School of Medicine— Resource for Tumor Tissue and Data
	Mount Sinai School of Medicine—Manhattan HIV Bank
	Mount Sinai School of Medicine of CUNY—Brain Bank Core
	New York Multiple Sclerosis Consortium
	New York University Medical Center—Breast Cancer Specimen Bank
	The Research Institute on Addictions—Biologic Specimen Bank
	Sloan-Kettering Institute
	The Taub Center for Alzheimer's Disease Research Tissue Bank
	Tumor Bank Facility at Columbia-Presbyterian Medical Center's Herbert Irving Comprehensive Cancer Center
	University Center of Downstate Medical Center—Tissue Bank for Research on HIV-associated Malignancies
	University of Rochester Alzheimer's Disease Center
	Weill Medical College of Cornell University—Tissue Culture Core
North Carolina	Duke University—Breast Cancer Specimen Bank
	Duke University—Kathleen Price Bryan Brain Bank
	UNC Lineberger Comprehensive Cancer Center—SPORE in Breast Cancer
Ohio	GOG Tissue Bank
	Ohio State University Comprehensive Cancer Center—Tissue Procurement Shared Resource
Oklahoma	Oklahoma City VA Medical Center—Cell and Tissue Bank for Marker Studies of Diseases of the Bladder, Prostate, Kidney, Lung, and Breast
Oregon	Kaiser Permanente Center for Health Research
Pennsylvania	Fox Chase Network Breast Cancer Risk Registry
	National Disease Research Interchange
	National Surgical Adjuvant Breast and Bowel Project (NSABP)
	Pittsburgh VA Medical Center—Pittsburgh Cancer Institute Serum Bank and Tissue Bank
	Pittsburgh VA Medical Center—Tissue Banking for Early Detection Research Network
	RTOG Tumor Tissue Repository
	University of Pennsylvania, Dept. of Microbiology—Brain Tissue Bank
	University of Pennsylvania—Breast Cancer Specimen Bank
	University of Pittsburgh Medical Center—Western Genitourinary Tissue Bank
	University of Pittsburgh—Human Brain Bank
Tennessee	Nashville VA Medical Center—Human Gastrointestinal Tumor Bank

Texas	Alzheimer's Disease Research Center at Baylor College of Medicine
	Baylor College of Medicine—Collection of DNA/RNA Tissue Repository for Neurodegenerative Disorders
	Baylor College of Medicine—Prostate SPORE
	National Psoriasis Tissue Bank
	San Antonio SPORE—Familial Breast Cancer Registry and Gene Bank
	San Antonio SPORE—National Breast Cancer Tissue Resource
	San Antonio VA Medical Center—Prostate Cancer Tumor Bank
	University of Texas M.D. Anderson Cancer Center—Tissue Core Facility at the Oral Cancer Research Center
	University of Texas M.D. Anderson Cancer Center—Tissue Procurement and Banking Facility
	University of Texas Southwestern's Medical Center—Tissue Procurement Core
Utah	Salt Lake City VA Medical Center—Regional Tumor Bank
Washington	LifeSpan BioSciences, Inc.
	University of Washington Alzheimer's Disease Research Center
	University of Washington—Center for Ecogenetics and Environmental Health
	University of Washington—Breast Cancer Database and Biologic Resource Bank
	University of Washington—International Registry of Werner Syndrome/Cell Bank
Wisconsin	Medical College of Wisconsin—Wisconsin's Alzheimer's Disease Brain Tissue Bank

TUMOR REGISTRIES BY STATE

California	California Tumor Tissue Registry Loma Linda University School of Medicine Dept. of Pathology 11021 Campus Ave., AH 335 Loma Linda, CA 92350 Ph. 909-558-4788 Fax: 909-558-0188 http://www.llu.edu/llu.cttr
	California Cancer Registry P.O. Box 942732, MS #592 Sacramento, CA 94234 Ph. 916-327-4663 Fax: 916-327-4657 http://www.ccrcal.org
	Cancer Registry of Central California 1625 E. Shaw Ave., Suite 155 Fresno, CA 93710 Ph. 559-274-4550 Fax: 559-221-1821
	Tri-Counties Regional Cancer Registry 345 Camino Del Remedio, Rm. M340 Santa Barbara, CA 03110 Ph. 805-681-5136 Fax: 805-681-5159
	Cancer Registry of Northern California 1560 Humboldt Rd., Suite 4 Chico, CA 95928 Ph. 530-345-2483 Fax: 530-345-3214
Colorado	Colorado Central Cancer Registry Colorado Dept. of Public Health and Environment Prevention Programs Division 4300 Cherry Creek Dr. South PPD-CR-A5 Denver, CO 80222 Ph. 303-692-2540 Fax: 303-782-0095 http://sedac.ciesin.org/ozone/regs/colorado.html

Connecticut	Tumor Registry Section Dept. of Public Health 410-450 Capitol Ave. Hartford, CT 06134
	Hartford Hospital Cancer Registry 80 Seymour St. Hartford, CT 06102 Ph. 860-545-5555 http://www.harthosp.org/cancer/registry
Florida	Florida Cancer Data System Division of Cancer Prevention and Control University of Miami School of Medicine P.O. Box 016960 Miami, FL 33101 Ph. 305-243-4600 Fax: 305-243-4871 http://fcds.med.miami.edu/
Georgia	Tumor Registry Phoebe Putney Memorial Hospital 417 Third Ave. Albany, GA 31703 Ph. 912-883-1800
	Georgia Comprehensive Cancer Registry Georgia Division of Public Health 2 Peachtree St., N.W. Atlanta, GA 30303 http://www.ph.dhr.state.ga.us/org/ cancercontrolsection.cancerregistry.htm
Hawaii	The Hawaii Tumor Registry 1236 Lauhala St. Honolulu, Hawaii 96813 Ph. 808-586-9750 Fax: 808-587-0024 http://www.planet-hawaii.com/htr
Idaho	Cancer Data Registry of Idaho 802 W. Bannock Suite 500 P.O. Box 1278 Boise, ID 83701 http://www.idcancer.org
Illinois	Illinois State Cancer Registry Illinois Dept. of Public Health 535 W. Jefferson St. Springfield, IL 62761 Ph. 217-782-4977 Fax: 217-782-3987 http://hometown.aol.com/epistudies/cancer/index.htm

Indiana	Tumor Registry at St. Joseph's Medical Center 801 E. LaSalle South Bend, IN 46617 Ph. 219-237-7111 Fax: 219-239-4024
Iowa	State Health Registry of Iowa University of Iowa Iowa City, Iowa 52242 Ph. 319-335-8609 http://www.uiowa.edu/~vpr/research/organize/healthreg.htm
Kansas	Kansas Cancer Registry 5028 Robinson Hall 3901 Rainbow Blvd. Kansas City, KS 66160 Ph. 913-588-4730 http://www.kumc.edu/som/kcr
Kentucky	Kentucky Cancer Registry 306 Davis-Mills Building 800 Rose St. Lexington, KY 40536 Ph. 606-257-4582 Fax: 305-243-4871 http://www.kcr.uky.edu
Louisiana	Louisiana Tumor Registry Dept. of Public Health & Preventive Medicine Louisiana Tumor Registry Suite 900 Box 106 1600 Canal St. New Orleans, LA 70112 Ph. 504-568-4716 Fax: 504-568-2493 New Orleans Regional Tumor Registry P.O. Box 60630 New Orleans, LA 70160 Ph. 504-568-2616 Fax: 504-599-1377 Baton Rouge Regional Tumor Registry 4950 Essen Lane Baton Rouge, LA 70809 Ph. 225-767-0430 Fax: 225-767-4742 Southeast Louisiana Regional Cancer P.O. Box 60630 New Orleans, LA 70160 Ph. 504-568-2616 Fax: 504-599-1377

Acadiana Tumor Registry
705 E. Saint Mary Blvd.
Lafayette, LA 70503
Ph. 318-237-5398
Fax: 318-235-9436

S.W. Louisiana Regional Tumor Registry
524 South Ryan St.
Lake Charles, LA 70601
Ph. 318-491-7790
Fax: 318-430-5471

Central Louisiana Regional Tumor Registry
Northeast Louisiana University
700 University Ave.
CNSB Room 221
Monroe, LA 71209
Ph. 318-342-1820
Fax: 318-342-1824

Northwest Louisiana Regional Cancer Registry
LSU Medical Center—Shreveport
Section Cancer Prevention & Control
P.O. Box 33932
Shreveport, LA 71130
Ph. 318-675-7660
Fax: 318-675-7600

North Louisiana Regional Tumor Registry
Northeast Louisiana University
700 University Ave.
CNSB Room 226
Monroe, LA 71209
Ph. 318-342-1840
Fax: 318-342-1824

Maine

Central Maine Medical Center Cancer Registry
300 Main St.
Lewiston, ME 04240
Ph. 207-795-2496
http://www2.cmmc.org/cmmc/cancercare/registry.html

Maryland

National Familial Brain Tumor Registry
The Johns Hopkins Oncology Center
600 N. Wolfe St., Room 132
Baltimore, MD 21287
Ph. 410-955-0227

National Familial Lung Cancer Registry
The Johns Hopkins University School of Hygiene and Public Health
615 N. Wolfe St., Room 6309
Baltimore, MD 21205
Ph. 410-614-1910
Fax: 410-955-0863
http://www.path.jhu.edu/nfltr.html

Massachusetts

Massachusetts Cancer Registry
250 Washington St.
Boston, MA 02108

MGH Cancer Data Registry
32 Fruit St.
Boston, MA 02114
Ph. 617-726-8646
Fax: 617-724-3013
http://cancer.mgh.harvard.edu/tumreg/tumreg.htm

New Hampshire   Tumor Registry at the Cheshire
Medical Center
580 Court St.
Keene, NH 03431
Ph. 603-352-4111

New Jersey   New Jersey State Cancer Registry
3635 Quaker Bridge Rd.
CN 369
Trenton, NJ 08625
Ph. 609-588-3500
Fax: 609-588-7431
http://www.ker.state.nj.us/health/cancer/njscr1b.htm

New York   Metropolitan New York Registry
NYU Medical Center, Dept. of Environmental Medicine
341 E. 25th St., Room 209
New York, NY 10010
Ph. 212-263-5964
Fax: 212-263-8570
http://www.med.nyu.edu/Biostat-Epi/mnyr.htm

North Carolina   Tumor Registry at Duke University's Comprehensive Cancer Center
3100 Tower Blvd., Suite 1602
Box 3153 Medical Center
Durham, NC 27710
Ph. 919-419-7900

North Carolina Cancer Registry
State Center for Health Statistics
1908 Mail Service Center
Raleigh, NC 27699
Ph. 919-715-9728
http://www.schs.state.nc.us/SCHS/about/branches/ccr.html

Ohio   American Academy of Pediatrics
Prepubertal Testicular Tumor Registry
9500 Euclid Ave.
Cleveland, OH 44195
Fax: 216-444-0088

Oregon   Oregon State Cancer Registry
Health Promotion and Chronic Disease Prevention
800 N.E. Oregon St., Suite 368
Portland, OR 97232
Ph. 503-713-4858
Fax: 503-713-4848
http://www.orcpr.org/oscar.html

Rhode Island	Rhode Island Cancer Registry Rhode Island Dept. of Health 3 Capitol Hill Providence, RI 02908 Ph. 401-453-8424 http://www.health.state.ri.us/canrep.htm
South Carolina	Savannah River Region Cancer Incidence Registry Medical University of South Carolina Biometry and Epidemiology 550 MUSC Complex Suite 1133 Charleston, SC 29425 Ph. 843-876-1142 Fax: 843-876-1143 http://www.musc.edu/srrhis/
	Hollings Cancer Center High Risk Lung Cancer Registry Medical University of South Carolina 171 Ashley Ave. Charleston, SC 29425 Ph. 843-792-9074 http:/hcc.musc.edu/lungreg
Tennessee	International Pediatric Adrenocortical Tumor Registry Peds/Hem/Onc St. Jude Children's Research Hospital 332 N. Lauderdale Memphis, TN 38105 http://www.stjude.org/ipactr/objectives.htm
Texas	Familial Brain Tumor Registry University of Texas M.D. Anderson Cancer Center Dept. of Epidemiology, Box 189 1515 Holcombe Blvd. Houston, TX 77340 Ph. 800-248-4856 Fax: 713-792-8261
	Medical Informatics—Tumor Registry University of Texas M.D. Anderson Cancer Center Dept. of Epidemiology, Box 189 1515 Holcombe Blvd. Houston, TX 77030 Ph. 713-792-6630 Fax: 713-792-6401
	Texas Cancer Data Center 1515 Holcombe Blvd. HMB 223 Houston, TX 77030 Ph. 713-792-2277 Fax: 713-794-1951 http://www.txcancer.org

Vermont	Vermont Cancer Registry Vermont Dept. of Health P.O. Box 70 Burlington, VT 05402 Ph. 802-865-7749 http://www.senate.gov/~leahy/bcreg.htm
Virginia	Virginia Cancer Registry Virginia Dept. of Health Office of Epidemiology Division of Surveillance and Investigation P.O. Box 2448, Rm. 114 Richmond, VA 23218 Ph. 804-786-1668 Fax: 804-371-4061 http://www.vdh.state.va.us/epi/ver.htm
Washington	Washington State Cancer Registry Washington State Dept. of Health 1112 S.E. Quince St. P.O. Box 47890 Olympia, WA 98504 http://www.doh.wa.gov/ehspl/epidemiology/wscr1.htm
Wisconsin	Wisconsin Cancer Reporting System Dept. of Health and Family Services 1 W. Wilson St. Madison, WI 53702 Ph. 608-266-1865 http://www.dhfs.state.wi.us/wcrs/object.htm
Wyoming	Wyoming Cancer Surveillance Program Wyoming Dept. of Health Hathaway Building Cheyenne, WY 82002 Ph. 307-777-7951 Fax: 307-777-5402 http://wdhfs.state.wy.us/cancer

ALPHABETICAL LISTING BY STATE OF LONGITUDINAL STUDIES AND RESEARCH PROJECTS THAT SIMULTANEOUSLY CREATE TISSUE BANKS

California	AIDS-Malignancy Clinical Trials Consortium (University of Southern California)
	Epidemiology of EBV-Defined Hodgkin's Disease (Northern California Cancer Center)
	Exogenous Toxicants and Genetic Susceptibility in Amyotrophic Lateral Sclerosis (Stanford University)
Colorado	Smoking Cessation Program for Patients Enrolled in SPORE Projects (Denver VAMC)
District of Columbia	Markers for Malignant Progression in Prostate Cancer (Georgetown University)
Georgia	National Health and Nutrition Examination Survey (CDC)
Kentucky	The Nun Study (University of Kentucky)
Louisiana	Bogalusa Heart Study (Louisiana State University Medical Center) http://www.mcl.tulane.edu/cardiohealth.bog.htm
Maryland	Baltimore Longitudinal Study of Aging (National Institutes of Aging)
	National Institute of Child Health and Human Development (research projects on pregnancy, delivery, and child development–related issues)
	The National Institutes of Health Women's Health Initiative (Tissue samples stored in Maryland; Clinical Coordinating Center in Seattle, Washington)
Massachusetts	Framingham Heart Study
	Physicians' Health Study (Brigham and Women's Hospital)
	Women's Health Study (Brigham and Women's Hospital)
Minnesota	Prostate Cancer Intervention versus Observation Trial (Minneapolis VAMC)
New Jersey	Prospective Randomized Study of Adjuvant Chemotherapy versus Vinorelbine and Cisplatin in Completely Resected NSCLC with Comparison Tumor Marker Evaluation (East Orange VAMC)
New York	Blood Test to Predict Prognosis in Patients with Gynecologic Cancer: Plasma Assay of GLB and GLB:TIMP-1 Complexes (Northport VAMC)
	Lifetime Alcohol Exposure and Breast Cancer Risk (State University of New York at Buffalo)

North Carolina	Molecular Basis of Split Hand/Foot Malformation (University of North Carolina)
Ohio	Molecular Epidemiology of Breast Cancer (Case Western Reserve University)
Pennsylvania	Case-Control Study of Hodgkin's Disease in Children (University of Pittsburgh)
	Genetics of Familial Polycystic Ovary Syndrome (Milton S. Hershey Medical Center)
	The Role of IL-1 Cytokines in Colorectal Cancer (Pittsburgh VAMC)
Tennessee	Pulmonary Hypertension—Mechanisms and Family Registry (Vanderbilt University Hospital)
Texas	Tissue and Biological Correlations of Soft Tissue Carcinoma (University of Texas M.D. Anderson Cancer Center)
Washington	Human Conceptual Tissue: Characterization for Transplantation
	Markers for Differentiated Diagnosis and Virulence of Prostate Cancer (Seattle VAMC)

TRANSPLANT ORGAN AND TISSUE BANKS BY STATE

Alabama

Alabama Community Blood Bank
(LifeSouth Community Blood Centers)
386 W. Orange Rd.
Birmingham, AL 35209
Ph. 205-943-6000
Fax: 205-943-6003
http://www.crbs.org

Alabama Eye Bank
500 Robert Jemison Rd.
Birmingham, AL 35209
Ph. 800-423-78101
http://www.uab.edu/eye/eyebank3.html

Alabama Organ Center
301 S. 20th St., Suite 1001
Birmingham, AL 35233-2033
Ph. 800-252-3677
Fax: 205-731-9250
http://www.uab.edu/aoc/

Alabama Tissue Center
855 THT, 1900 University Blvd.
Birmingham, AL 35294
Ph. 205-934-4314
Fax: 205-934-9219

Alaska

Blood Bank of Alaska, Inc.
400 Laurel St.
Anchorage, Alaska 99508
Ph. 907-563-3110
http://www.customcpu.com/np/bba/
default.htm

Arizona

Donor Network of Arizona
3877 N. 7th St., Suite 200
Phoenix, AZ 85014
Ph. 602-222-2200
Fax: 602-222-2202
http://www.donor-network.org

United Blood Services
6220 E. Oak St.
P.O. Box 1541
Scottsdale, AZ 85252
Ph. 602-431-9500
Fax: 602-675-5767
http://aztec.asu.edu/blood

Arkansas

Arkansas Regional Organ Recovery Agency
1100 N. University, Suite 200
Little Rock, AR 77207-6344
Ph. 501-224-2623
Fax: 501-372-6279

California

American Red Cross Tissue Services
Western Area
3535 Hyland Ave.
Costa Mesa, CA 92626
Ph. 714-708-1300
Fax: 714-708-1331

Blood Bank of the Redwoods
2324 Bethards Dr.
Santa Rosa, CA 95405
Ph. 707-545-1222
Fax: 707-575-8178
http://bbr.org

Blood Centers of the Pacific
270 Masonic Ave.
San Francisco, CA 94118
Ph. 415-567-6400
Fax: 415-921-6430
http://www.citysearch.com/sfo/bloodcenter

CA Transplant Donor Network
55 Francisco St., Suite 510
San Francisco, CA 94133
Ph. 415-837-5888
Fax: 415-837-5880

Central California Blood Center
3445 N. First St.
Fresno, CA 93726
Ph. 559-224-2900
Fax: 559-225-1602
http://www.cencalblood.org/default02.htm

Community Tissue Service
3445 N. First St.
Fresno, CA 93726
Ph. 800-201-8477
Fax: 559-229-7217

Cord Blood Registry
1200 Bayhill Dr.
Suite 301
San Bruno, CA 94066
Ph. 888-267-3256
http://www.cordblood.com

Delta Blood Bank
65 N. Commerce St.
P.O. Box 800
Stockton, CA 95201
Ph. 209-943-3830
Fax: 209-462-0221

Doheny Eye and Tissue Transplant Bank
1450 San Pablo St., Suite 3600
Los Angeles, CA 90033
Ph. 213-223-0333
Fax: 213-342-7155

Doheny Eye and Tissue Transplant Bank of Central Coast
5553 Hollister Ave., Suite 4
Goleta, CA 93117
Ph. 805-681-3224
Fax: 805-681-3226

Golden State Donor Service
1760 Creekside Oaks Dr., Suite 160
Sacramento, CA 95833-3632
Ph. 916-567-1600
Fax: 916-567-8300

Houchin Community Blood Bank
2600 G St.
Eureka, CA 93301
Ph. 805-327-8541
Fax: 805-323-7304

Northern California Community Blood Bank
2524 Harrison Ave.
Eureka, CA 95501
Ph. 707-443-8004
Fax: 707-443-8007

Northern California Transplant Bank
2593 Kerner Blvd.
San Rafael, CA 94901
Ph. 800-922-3100
Fax: 415-455-9015

Orange County Eye & Tissue Bank
801 N. Tustin Ave., #102
Santa Ana, CA 92705
Ph. 714-550-1022
Fax: 714-550-9964

OTAC of Southern California
3665 Ruffin Rd., Suite 120
San Diego, CA 92123-1871
Ph. 619-292-8750
Fax: 619-560-5945

Regional OPA of Southern California
10920 Wilshire Blvd., Suite 910
Los Angeles, CA 90024
Ph. 310-206-0222
Fax: 310-825-5512

Sacramento Medical Foundation Blood Center
1625 Stockton Blvd.
Sacramento, CA 95816
Ph. 916-456-1500
Fax: 916-739-8219

San Diego Blood Bank
440 Upas St.
San Diego, CA 92103
Ph. 619-296-6393
Fax: 619-296-0126
http://www.sandiegobloodbank.org

Sierra Eye and Tissue Donor Services
1700 Alhambra Blvd., Suite 112
Sacramento, CA 95816
Ph. 916-456-1450
Fax: 916-456-3731

Southern CA Organ Procurement Center
2200 W. Third St., 2nd Floor
Los Angeles, CA 90057
Ph. 213-413-6219
Fax: 213-413-5373

United Blood Services
1756 Eastman Ave., Suite 104
P.O. Box 760
Ventura, CA 93002
Ph. 805-654-1600
Fax: 805-658-6527

Colorado

AlloSource
8085 E. Harvard Ave.
Denver, CO 80231
Ph. 303-755-7775
Fax: 303-755-7111

Bonfils Memorial Blood Center
717 Yosemite Circle
Denver, CO 80230
Ph. 303-341-4000
Fax: 303-340-2927

Donor Alliance, Inc. (Mile High Transplant Bank)
3773 Cherry Creek N. Dr., Suite 601
Denver, CO 80209
Ph. 800-448-4644
Fax: 303-321-0366

Rocky Mountain Lions Eye Bank
695 S. Colorado Blvd., Suite 320
Denver, CO 80246
Ph. 800-444-7479
Fax: 303-778-0428
http://www.corneas.org

Rocky Mountain Multiple Sclerosis
Center Tissue Bank
701 E. Hampden Ave.
Suite 420
Englewood, CO 80110
Ph. 303-788-7806
http://www.swedmc.com:80/msc/tissue.htm

Rocky Mountain Tissue Bank
2993 S. Peoria St., Suite 390
Aurora, CO 80014
Ph. 303-337-3330
Fax: 303-337-9383

Connecticut

North East OPO and Tissue Bank
P.O. Box 5037
Hartford, CT 06102
Ph. 800-545-2256
Fax: 860-545-4153

Delaware

Blood Bank of Delaware
100 Hygeia Dr.
Newark, DE 19713
Ph. 302-737-8406
Fax: 302-737-8233

Florida

Central Florida Blood and Tissue Bank
32 W. Gore St.
Orlando, FL 32806
Ph. 407-849-6100
Fax: 407-649-8517
http://www.cfbb.org

Central Florida Lions Eye & Tissue Bank, Inc.
5523 W. Cypress St., Suite 100
Tampa, FL 33607
Ph. 813-289-1200
http://www.lionseyebank.com/home.html

Community Blood Centers of South Florida
1700 N. State Rd. 7
Ft. Lauderdale, FL 33313
Ph. 954-735-9600
Fax: 954-735-2839
http://www.cbcsf.org

Florida Blood Services
3602 Spectrum Blvd.
P.O. Box 2125
Tampa, FL 33601
Ph. 813-632-5433
Fax: 813-903-1177
http://www.fbsblood.org

Florida Georgia Blood Alliance
536 W. 10th St.
Jacksonville, FL 32206
Ph. 904-353-8263
Fax: 904-358-7111
http://www.fgba.org

LifeLink Tissue Bank
8510 Sunstate St.
Tampa, FL 33634
Ph. 800-683-2400
Fax: 813-888-9419

Lifelink of Florida
2111 Swann Ave.
Tampa, FL 33606-2423
Ph. 813-253-2640
Fax: 813-251-1819

Lifelink of Southwest Florida
12573 New Brittany Blvd., #10
Fort Myers, FL 33907
Ph. 813-936-2772

LifeSouth Community Blood Centers
1221 N.W. 13th St.
Gainesville, FL 32601
Ph. 352-334-1000
Fax: 352-334-1066
http://www.crbs.org

Manatee Community Blood Center
216 Manatee Ave., E.
Bradenton, FL 34208
Ph. 941-746-7195
Fax: 941-748-1711

Medical Eye Bank of Florida
22 W. Lake Beauty Dr.
Orlando, FL 32806
Ph. 407-422-2020
Fax: 407-425-7262
http://www.castlegate.net/MEBFL/index.htm

North Florida Lions Eye Bank
1235 San Marco Blvd., Suite 201
Jacksonville, FL 32207
Ph. 800-822-4483
Fax: 904-346-0444

Northwest Florida Blood Center
2201 N. 9th Ave.
Pensacola, FL 32503
Ph. 850-434-2535
Fax: 850-469-9514

OPO at the University of Florida
Shands Hospital Dept. of Surgery
Box 100286
Gainesville, FL 32610
Ph. 352-395-0632
Fax: 352-338-9886

Sarasota Community Blood Bank
1760 Mound St.
Sarasota, FL 34236
Ph. 941-954-1600
Fax: 941-951-2629
http://www.sarasota-online.com/scbb

Southeastern Community Blood Center
1731 Riggins Rd.
Tallahassee, FL 32503
Ph. 850-877-7181
Fax: 850-469-7435
http://scbcinfo.org

Translife
2501 N. Orange Ave., Suite 40
Orlando, FL 32804
Ph. 407-897-5560

TransLife/Florida Hospital
2501 N. Orange Ave., Suite 40
Orlando, FL 32804
Ph. 407-897-5560
Fax: 407-897-5574

University of Miami
Dept. of Ortho Rehab Tissue Bank
P.O. Box 016960 (R-12)
1600 N.W. 10th Ave.
Miami, FL 33101
Ph. 305-243-6786
Fax: 305-243-4622

University of Miami OPO
1150 N.W. 14th St., Suite 208
Miami, FL 33136
Ph. 305-548-7622
Fax: 305-243-7628

Georgia

Atlanta LifeSouth Community Blood Centers
2215 Cheshire Bridge Rd.
Atlanta, GA 30324
Ph. 404-329-1994
Fax: 404-329-1465
http://www.crbs.org

LifeLink of Georgia
3715 Northside Parkway Building 100
Suite 300
Atlanta, GA 30327
Ph. 404-266-8884
Fax: 404-266-0592

Shepeard Community Blood Center
1533 Wrightsboro Rd.
Augusta, GA 30904
Ph. 706-737-4551
Fax: 706-733-5214
http://www.shepeardblood.com

South Georgia Branch of Southeastern Community Blood Center
2705 E. Pinetree Blvd., Suite 4
Thomasville, GA 31792
Ph. 912-228-9980
http://www.scbcinfo.org

Hawaii

Blood Bank of Hawaii
2043 Dillingham Blvd.
Honolulu, HI 96819
Ph. 808-845-9966
Fax: 808-848-4737

Hawaii Lions Eye Bank
P.O. Box 2783
Honolulu, HI 96803
Ph. 808-536-7416
Fax: 808-528-5032
http://www.eyebank.org

Organ Donor Center of Hawaii
1000 Bishop St., Suite 302
Honolulu, HI 96813
Ph. 808-599-7630
Fax: 808-599-7631

Illinois

Bromenn Watson-Gailey Eye Bank
Virginia at Franklin
Normal, IL 61761
Ph. 800-548-4703
Fax: 309-454-3486

Central Illinois Community Blood Bank
1134 S. Seventh St.
Springfield, IL 62703
Ph. 217-753-1530
Fax: 217-753-0689
http://www.fgi.net/~bloodbnk

Community Blood Services of Illinois
1408 W. University Ave.
Urbana, IL 61801
Ph. 217-367-2202
Fax: 217-367-6403

Heartland Blood Centers
1200 N. Highland Ave.
Aurora, IL 60506
Ph. 630-892-7055
Fax: 630-892-4590

Illinois Eye Bank
800 S. Wells St., Suite 185
Chicago, IL 60607
Ph. 800-548-4703
Fax: 312-431-3433

LifeSource
1205 N. Milwaukee Ave.
Glenview, IL 60025
Ph. 847-803-7830
Fax: 847-803-7685
http://www.itxm.org

Regional Organ Bank of Illinois
800 S. Wells, Suite 190
Chicago, IL 60607-4529
Ph. 312-431-3600
Fax: 312-803-7643
http://www.robi.org

Indiana

American Red Cross Tissue Services
Central States Area
1000 C Airport North Office
Fort Wayne, IN 46825
Ph. 219-497-7159
Fax: 219-489-6994

Central Indiana Regional Blood Center Tissue Bank
3450 N. Meridian St.
Indianapolis, IN 46208
Ph. 317-926-2381
Fax: 317-927-1724
http://www.donor-link.org

Clarion Health Eye and Tissue Bank
1701 N. Senate Blvd.
BG 54
Indianapolis, IN 46206
Ph. 317-929-2333
Fax: 317-929-8216

Indiana Lions Eye Bank
702 Rotary Circle, Room 146
Indianapolis, IN 46202
Ph. 317-274-8527
Fax: 317-274-2180

Indiana OPO
719 Indiana Ave., Suite 100
Indianapolis, IN 46202
Ph. 317-685-0389
Fax: 317-685-1687

Iowa

Blood Center of Central Iowa
1050 Seventh St.
Des Moines, IA 50314
Ph. 515-288-0276
Fax: 515-288-0833
http://www.bloodonor.org

Iowa Statewide OPO
2732 Northgate Dr.
Iowa City, IA 52245
Ph. 800-831-4131
Fax: 319-337-6105

Mercy Medical Center Surgical Bone Bank
710 10th St. S.E.
Cedar Rapids, IA 52403
Ph. 319-398-6756
Fax: 319-398-6229

Mississippi Valley Regional Blood Center
3425 E. Locust St.
Davenport, IA 52803
Ph. 319-359-5401
Fax: 319-359-8603

Siouxland Community Blood Bank
1019 Jones St.
P.O. Box 1566
Sioux City, IA 51102
Ph. 712-252-2534
Fax: 606-233-4166

Southeast Iowa Blood Center
1005 E. Pennsylvania
Ottumwa, IA 52501
Ph. 515-682-8149
Fax: 515-682-6017

Kansas

Midwest Organ Bank
1900 W. 47th Place, Suite 400
Westwood, KS 66205
Ph. 913-262-1666
Fax: 913-262-5130

Wichita Eye Bank
3306 E. Central Ave.
Wichita, KS 67208
Ph. 800-393-3008
Fax: 316-688-7390
http://www2.southwind.net/~gsbryan

Kentucky

Central Kentucky Blood Center
330 Waller Ave.
Lexington, KY 40504
Ph. 606-276-2534
Fax: 606-233-4166

Kentucky Lions Eye Bank
301 E. Muhammad Ali Blvd.
Louisville, KY 40202
Ph. 502-852-5466
Fax: 502-852-7298
http://athena.louisville.edu/medschool/ophthalmology/kleb.htm

Kentucky Organ Donor Affiliates
106 E. Broadway
Louisville, KY 40202
Ph. 502-581-9511
Fax: 502-589-5157

Western Kentucky Regional Blood Center
3015 Hartford Rd.
Owensboro, KY 42301
Ph. 270-684-9296
Fax: 270-684-4901

Louisiana

Blood Center for Southeast Louisiana
312 S. Galvez St.
New Orleans, LA 70119
Ph. 504-524-1322
Fax: 504-592-2694
http://www.thebloodcenter.org

Lifeshare Blood Centers
1455 Wilkinson St.
Shreveport, LA 71103
Ph. 318-222-7770
Fax: 318-222-8886

Louisiana OPA
3501 N. Causeway Blvd., Suite 940
Metairie, LA 70002
Ph. 504-837-3355
Fax: 504-837-3587

Southern Transplant Services, Inc.
Houma Medical Center
3901 Houma Blvd., Plaza 2, #405
Metairie, LA 70006
Ph. 504-454-7998
Fax: 504-885-7873

United Blood Services
1503 Bertrand Dr.
P.O. Box 3362
Lafayette, LA 70502
Ph. 318-235-5433
Fax: 318-232-5352
http://aztec.asu.edu/blood

Maryland

Blood Bank of Delaware
1309 Mt. Hermon Rd.
Salisbury, MD 21801
Ph. 410-749-4161
Fax: 410-749-7303

Medical Eye Bank of Maryland
Washington Eye Bank
815 Park Ave.
Baltimore, MD 21201
Ph. 410-752-3800
Fax: 410-545-4455

Transplant Resource Center of Maryland
1540 Caton Center Dr., Suite R
Baltimore, MD 21227
Ph. 410-242-7000
Fax: 410-242-1871

Massachusetts

New England Cord Blood Bank
665 Beacon St., Suite 302
Boston, MA 02215
Ph. 800-700-CORD
http://www.cordbloodbank.com/overview.htm

New England Eye & Tissue Transplant Bank
50 Staniford St., 4th Floor
Boston, MA 02114
Ph. 617-523-3937
Fax: 617-523-2364

New England Organ Bank
One Gateway Center
Newton, MA 02158
Ph. 800-446-6362
Fax: 617-244-8755
http://www.neob.org

Michigan

Michigan Community Blood Centers
1036 Fuller Ave., N.E.
P.O. Box 1704
Grand Rapids, MI 49501
Ph. 616-774-2300
Fax: 616-776-1891
http://miblood.org

Michigan Eye Bank
1000 Wall St.
Ann Arbor, MI 48105
Ph. 800-247-7250
Fax: 734-936-0020
http://www.mebtc.org

Transplantation Society of Michigan
2203 Platt Rd.
Ann Arbor, MI 48104
Ph. 313-973-1577
Fax: 313-973-3133

University of Michigan Skin Bank
1500 E. Medical Center Dr.
Rm. 1A435-UH, Box 0033
Ann Arbor, MI 48109
Ph. 313-936-9673
Fax: 313-936-9657

Minnesota

American Red Cross Tissue Services
North Central Region
100 S. Robert St.
St. Paul, MN 55107
Ph. 800-847-7838
Fax: 651-290-8925

Lifesource, Upper Midwest OPO, Inc.
2550 University Ave. W.,
Suite 315 S.
St. Paul, MN 55114-1904
Ph. 612-603-7800
Fax: 612-603-7801

Memorial Blood Centers of Minnesota
2304 Park Ave.
Minneapolis, MN 55404
Ph. 612-871-3300
Fax: 612-871-1359
http://www.mbcm.org

Mississippi

Mississippi Blood Services
1995 Lakeland Dr.
Jackson, MS 39216
Ph. 601-981-3232
Fax: 601-984-3783

Mississippi Organ Recovery Agency
12 River Bend Place, Suite B
Jackson, MS 39208
Ph. 601-933-1000
Fax: 601-933-1006

United Blood Services
604 W. Eastern Blvd.
P.O. Box 2577
Tupelo, MS 38803
Ph. 601-842-8871
Fax: 601-680-9161
http://www.mississippi.net/~jrigdon/index.html

Missouri

Community Blood Center of Greater Kansas City
4040 Main St.
Kansas City, MO 64111
Ph. 816-753-4040
Fax: 816-968-4047
http://kcblood.org

Mid-America Transplant Association
1139 Olivette Executive Parkway
St. Louis, MO 63132-3205
Ph. 314-991-1661
Fax: 314-991-2805

Missouri Lions Eye Research Foundation
404 Portland St.
Columbia, MO 65201
Ph. 573-443-1471

St. Louis Cord Blood Bank
3662 Park Ave.
St. Louis, MO 63110
Ph. 314-268-2787
Fax: 314-268-4081
http://www.slu.edu/colleges/med/departments/pediatrics/cordbank/
moreinfo.html

Montana

United Blood Services
3000 7th Ave., N.
P.O. Box 1672
Billings, MT 64111
Ph. 816-248-9168
Fax: 406-248-1025
http://aztec.asu.edu/blood

Nebraska

Community Blood Bank of the Lancaster County Medical Society
2966 O St.
Lincoln, NE 68510
Ph. 402-474-1781
Fax: 402-474-5986
http://www.medlinc.com/lcms/bloodbnk

Nebraska Organ Retrieval System
4060 Vinton St., Suite 200
Omaha, NE 68105
Ph. 402-553-7952
Fax: 402-553-0933

Nevada

Nevada Donor Network
4580 S. Eastern Ave., Suite 33
Las Vegas, NV 89119
Ph. 702-796-9600
Fax: 702-796-4225

United Blood Services
6930 W. Charleston Blvd.
Las Vegas, NV 89117
Ph. 702-228-4483
Fax: 702-228-2374
http://www.unitedbloodservices.org

United Blood Services
1125 Terminal Way
Reno, NV 89502
Ph. 702-329-6451
Fax: 702-324-6480
http://aztec.asu.edu/blood

New Jersey

BioGenetics Corporation
1130 Rte. 22W, P.O. Box 1290
Mountainside, NJ 07092
Ph. 908-654-8836
Fax: 908-232-2114

Blood Center of New Jersey
45 S. Grove St.
East Orange, NJ 07018
Ph. 973-676-4700
Fax: 973-676-4933
http://www.bloodnj.org

Central New Jersey Blood Center
494 Sycamore Ave.
Shrewsbury, NJ 07702
Ph. 732-842-5750
Fax: 732-842-1617
http://www.cjbc.org

Community Blood Services
970 Linwood Ave. W.
Paramus, NJ 07652
Ph. 201-444-3900
Fax: 201-670-6174

Lions Eye Bank of New Jersey
DOC –1st Floor, 90 Bergen St.
Newark, NJ 07103
Ph. 973-972-2060
Fax: 973-972-2093

Musculoskeletal Transplant Foundation
Edison Corporate Center
125 May St., Suite 300
Edison, NJ 08837
Ph. 732-661-0202
Fax: 732-661-2297

New Jersey Organ and Tissue Sharing Network
841 Mountain Ave.
Springfield, NJ 07081
Ph. 800-SHARE-NJ
Fax: 201-379-5113
http://www.sharenj.org

Osteotech, Inc.
51 James Way
Eatontown, NJ 07724
Ph. 732-542-2800
Fax: 732-542-2906

Tutogen Medical, Inc.
1719 Route 10
Parsippany, NJ 07054
Ph. 973-359-8444
Fax: 973-359-8410

New Mexico

New Mexico Donor Program
2715 Broadbent Parkway, Suite J
Albuquerque, NM 87107
Ph. 505-843-7672
Fax: 505-343-1828

New Mexico Lions Eye Bank
303 San Mateo Blvd., Suite 103
Albuquerque, NM 87108
Ph. 505-266-3937
Fax: 505-266-5560

United Blood Services
1515 University Blvd., N.E.
P.O. Box 25445
Albuquerque, NM 87125
Ph. 505-843-6227
Fax: 505-247-8835
http://aztec.asu.edu/blood

New York

American Red Cross Tissue Services
Greater Northeast Region
636 S. Warren St.
Syracuse, NY 13202
Ph. 315-464-1300
Fax: 315-425-0471

Center for Donation and Transplant
218 Great Oaks Blvd.
Albany, NY 12208
Ph. 518-262-5606
Fax: 518-262-5427

Eye Bank for Sight Restoration, Inc.
120 Wall St., Fl. 3
New York, NY 10005
Ph. 212-742-9000

Idant Laboratories
350 5th Ave., Suite 7120
New York, NY 10118
Ph. 212-244-0555
Fax: 212-244-0806

New York Blood Center
150 Amsterdam Ave.
New York, NY 10023
Ph. 800-933-BLOOD
http://www.nybloodcenter.org

New York Organ Donor Network
475 Riverside Dr., Suite 1244
New York, NY 10115
Ph. 212-870-2240
Fax: 212-870-3299

Rochester Eye and Human Parts Bank
524 White Spruce Blvd.
Rochester, NY 14623
Ph. 800-568-4321
http://www.rehpb.org

University of Rochester Organ Procurement Program
Corporate Woods of Brighton
Bldg. 120, Suite 180
Rochester, NY 14623
Ph. 716-272-4930
Fax: 716-272-4956

Upstate New York Transplant Services
165 Genesee St., Suite 102
Buffalo, NY 14203
Ph. 716-853-6667
Fax: 716-853-6674

North Carolina

Carolina LifeCare
Medical Center Blvd.
Winston Salem, NC 27157
Ph. 910-777-3130
Fax: 910-777-3137

Carolina OPA
702 Johns Hopkins Dr.
Greenville, NC 27834
Ph. 919-957-0090
Fax: 919-757-0708

LifeShare of Carolinas
101 W. T. Harris Blvd., Suite 5302
P.O. Box 32861
Charlotte, NC 28232
Ph. 704-548-6850
Fax: 704-548-6851

North Dakota

United Blood Services
517 S. 7th St.
P.O. Box 2052
Bismarck, ND 58502
Ph. 701-258-4512
Fax: 701-223-0557
http://aztec.asu.edu/blood

United Blood Services
1320 1st Ave. N.
P.O. Box 2462
Fargo, ND 58108
Ph. 701-293-9453
Fax: 513-558-1300
http://aztec.asu.edu/blood

Ohio

Community Tissue Services Community Blood Center
349 S. Main St.
Dayton, OH 45402
Ph. 800-684-7783
Fax: 937-461-4225

Hoxworth Blood Center
University of Cincinnati Medical Ctr.
3130 Highland Ave., ML0055
Cincinnati, OH 45267
Ph. 513-558-1200
Fax: 513-558 1300
http://www.hoxworth.org

Life Connection of Ohio
1545 Holland Rd., Suite C
Maumee, OH 43537
Ph 419-893 4891

LifeBand
20600 Chagrin Blvd., Suite 350
Cleveland, OH 44122-5343
Ph. 216-752-5433
Fax: 216-751-4204

Lifeline of Ohio Organ Procurement
770 Kinnear Rd., Suite 200
Columbus, OH 43212
Ph. 614-291-5667
Fax: 614-291-0660

Lifeshare
105 Cleveland St.
Dayton, OH 45402
Ph. 440-322-5700
Fax: 440-323-6240

Lions Eye Bank of West Central Ohio
120 Ziegler St., Suite 100
Dayton, OH 45402
Ph. 937-223-4850
Fax: 937-223-1541

Mid-America Tissue Center, Inc.
2860 Lincoln Way E.
Massillon, OH 44646
Ph. 800-451-3587
Fax: 330-830-0628

Northwest Ohio Tissue Bank
2736 N. Holland-Sylvania Rd.
Toledo, OH 43615
Ph. 419-534-6930
Fax: 419-534-6928

Ohio Valley LifeCenter
2939 Vernon Place
Cincinnati, OH 45219
Ph. 513-558-5555
Fax: 513-558-5556

Ohio Valley Tissue and Skin Center
2939 Vernon Place
Cincinnati, OH 45219
Ph. 513-558-6400
Fax: 513-558-6440

Toledo Life Connection of Ohio
1545 Holland Rd., Suite C
Maumee, OH 43537
Ph. 419-893-4891
Fax: 419-893-1827

Oklahoma

American Red Cross Tissue Services
Southern Plains Area
601 N.E. 6th St.
Oklahoma City, OK 73104
Ph. 405-815-6530
Fax: 405-232-6819

McBride Clinic Bone Bank
1111 N. Dewey Ave.
Oklahoma City, OK 73103
Ph. 405-272-9671, ext. 456
Fax: 405-552-9355

Oklahoma Lions Eye Bank
608 Stanton L. Young
Oklahoma City, OK 73104
Ph. 405-271-5691
http://www.ionet.net/~oleb/lionseye.html

Oklahoma Organ Sharing Network
5801 N. Broadway, Suite 100
Oklahoma City, OK 73112
Ph. 405-840-5551
Fax: 405-840-9748

Plasma Alliance, Inc.
Oklahoma City, OK 73103
Ph. 405-521-9204

Sylvan N. Goldman Center Oklahoma Blood Institute
1001 N. Lincoln Blvd.
Oklahoma City, OK 73104
Ph. 405-297-5700
Fax: 405-297-5513

Oregon

Community Tissue Service
16361 N.E. Cameron Blvd.
Portland, OR 97230
Ph. 503-408-9394
Fax: 503-408-9395

Lane Memorial Blood Bank
2211 Willamette St.
Eugene, OR 97405
Ph. 541-484-9111
Fax: 541-484-6976
http://www.lanecountyblood.org

Lions Eye Bank of Oregon
1010 N.W. 22nd Ave, N144
Portland, OR 97210
Ph. 800-843-7793
Fax: 800-798-9040
http://www.orlions.org/cover.htm

Pacific Northwest Transplant Bank
2611 S.W. Third Ave., Suite 320
Portland, OR 97201-4952
Ph. 503-494-5560
Fax: 503-494-4725

Pennsylvania

The Center for Organ Recovery and Education Ride Park
204 Sigma Dr.
Pittsburgh, PA 15238
Ph. 412-963-3550
Fax: 412-963-3563

Central Pennsylvania Blood Bank
Libery Center Office Complex
8170 Adams Dr., Suite 100
Hummelstown, PA 17036
Ph. 717-566-6161
Fax: 717-566-7851

Community Blood Bank of Erie County
2646 Peach St.
Erie, PA 16508
Ph. 814-456-4206
Fax: 814-452-3966
http://www.eriebloodbank.org

Delaware Valley Transplant Program
2000 Hamilton St., Suite 201
Philadelphia, PA 19130
Ph. 610-543-6391
Fax: 215-557-9359

Institute for Transfusion Medicine
3636 Boulevard of the Allies
Pittsburgh, PA 17036
Ph. 800-310-9551
Fax: 412-209-7335
http://www.itxm.org

Lions Eye Bank of Northwest
Pennsylvania
5105 Richmond St.
Erie, PA 16509
Ph. 814-866-3545
Fax: 814-864-1875
http://www.unitedwayerie.org/eyebank

Miller Memorial Blood Center
1465 Valley Center Parkway
Bethlehem, PA 18017
Ph. 610-691-5850
Fax: 610-691-5423

Pennsylvania Regional Tissue Bank
814 Cedar Ave.
Scranton, PA 18505
Ph. 570-343-5433
Fax: 570-343-6993

University of Pennsylvania
Medical Center
Bone and Tissue Bank
3508 Market St., Suite 490
Philadelphia, PA 19104
Ph. 215-662-7488
Fax: 215-349-5083

Puerto Rico   LifeLink of Puerto Rico
Ponce de Leon Ave., Stop 36 1/2
Hato Rey, PR 00919
Ph. 809-758-2000

Rhode Island   Rhode Island Blood Center
405 Promenade St.
Providence, RI 02908
Ph. 401-453-8360
Fax: 401-453-8557
http://www.ribc.org

South Carolina   American Red Cross Tissue Services
Southeastern Area
2751 Bull St.
Columbia, SC 29201
Ph. 803-251-6150
Fax: 803-251-6105

Carolina-Georgia Blood Center
515 Grove Rd.
Greenville, SC 29605
Ph. 864-255-5000
Fax: 864-255-9514

South Carolina OPA
1064 Gardner Rd., #105
Charleston, SC 29407
Ph. 800-462-0755
Fax: 803-763-6393
http://www.midnet.sc.edu/scopa/scopa.htm

South Dakota

United Blood Services
2209 W. Omaha
P.O. Box 9608
Rapid City, SD 29605
Ph. 605-342-8585
Fax: 605-342-6662
http://aztec.asu.edu/blood

Tennessee

Blood Assurance, Inc.
700 E. Third St.
Chattanooga, TN 57709
Ph. 423-756-0966
Fax: 423-752-8460
http://www.bloodassurance.org

East Tennessee Lions Eye Bank
1924 Alcoa Highway, #U-26
Knoxville, TN 37920
Ph. 423-544-9625
Fax: 423-523-4869
http://www.korrnet.org/eyebank/index.html

Life Resources Regional Donor Center
2812 McKinley Rd.
Johnson City, TN 37604
Ph. 423-929-1638
Fax: 423-929-9598

Lifeblood/Mid South Regional Blood Center
1040 Madison Ave.
Memphis, TN 38104
Ph. 901-522-8585
Fax: 901-529-6393
http://www.lifeblood.com

Lifeline/West Tennessee Regional Blood Center
828 N. Parkway
Jackson, TN 38305
Ph. 901-427-4431
Fax: 901-422-4712

Mid-South Tissue Bank
4719 Spottswood
Memphis, TN 38117
Ph. 901-683-6566
Fax: 901-683-9910

Mid-South Transplant Foundation
956 Court Ave., Suite G-228
Memphis, TN 38163
Ph. 901-448-5910
Fax: 901-448-8126

Tennessee Donor Services
5908-D Toole Dr.
Knoxville, TN 37919
Ph. 423-588-5903
http://www.korrnet.org/donors

Tennessee Donor Services
DCI Donor Services
1714 Hayes St.
Nashville, TN 37203
Ph. 615-327-2247
Fax: 619-320-1655

Texas

Blood and Tissue Center of Central Texas
4300 N. Lamar Blvd.
Austin, TX 78756
Ph. 800-580-1121
Fax: 512-458-3859
http://www.austin.citysearch.com/E/V/AUSTX/0004/52/93/11.html

Carter Bloodcare
9000 Harry Hines Blvd.
Dallas, TX 75235
Ph. 214-351-8111
Fax: 214-351-9803

Coffee Memorial Blood Center
1915 Coulter Dr.
P.O. Box 3429
Amarillo, TX 79106
Ph. 806-358-4563
Fax: 806-358-2982

Community Tissue Services
708 S. Henderson St.
Suite A
Fort Worth, TX 76104
Ph. 817-882-2556
Fax: 817-882-2557

El Paso Regional Transplant Bank
4505 Alberta
El Paso, TX 79905
Ph. 915-544-6714
Fax: 915-544-5794

Great Plains Lions Eye Bank, Inc.
Dept. of Ophthalmology & Visual Sciences
School of Medicine
Texas Tech University Health Sciences Center
Lubbock, TX 79430
Ph. 806-743-2400
http://www.ttuhsc.edu/eye/defaultpage/main/EyeBank.htm

Gulf Coast Regional Blood Center
1400 La Concha Lane
Houston, TX 77054
Ph. 713-790-1200
Fax: 713-790-1007
http://www.giveblood.org

LifeCell, Corp.
3606 Research Forest Dr.
The Woodlands, TX 77381
Ph. 281-367-5368
Fax: 281-363-3360

LifeGift Organ Donation Center
5615 Kirby Dr., Suite 900
Houston, TX 77005
Ph. 713-523-4438
Fax: 713-737-8100

Lions Eye Bank of Central Texas
919 E. 32nd St.
Austin, TX 78705
Ph. 800-977-3937
Fax: 512-457-0658
http://www.io.com/~garycox/LEBCT.html

Nueces County Medical Society
Community Blood Bank
5025 Deepwood Circle
Corpus Christi, TX 78415
Ph. 361-855-4943
Fax: 361-855-2641

Shriners Hospital for Children
Burns Institute Galveston
301 University Blvd.
Galveston, TX 77555
Ph. 409-621-1366
Fax; 409-621-1390

South Texas Blood and Tissue Center
6211 IH-10 W.
San Antonio, TX 78201
Ph. 210-731-5565
Fax: 210-731-5505
http://www.bloodntissue.org

South Texas Organ Bank
8122 Datapoint Dr., Suite 1150
San Antonio, TX 78229
Ph. 210-614-7030
Fax: 210-614-2129

Southwest Organ Bank
3500 Maple Ave., Suite 800
Dallas, TX 75219
Ph. 214-821-1910
http://wg.dzn.com/swob/top.htm

Southwest Transplant Alliance
3710 Rawlins, #1100
Dallas, TX 75219
Ph. 800-788-8058
Fax: 214-827-8352
http://www.organ.org

Stewart Regional Blood Center
815 S. Baxter Ave.
Tyler, TX 75701
Ph. 903-535-5400
Fax: 903-535-5450

Texoma Regional Blood Center
3911 N. Texoma Parkway
Sherman, TX 75090
Ph. 903-893-4314
Fax: 903-893-8628

Transplant Services Center
University of Texas
Southwest Medical Center
5323 Harry Hines Blvd. MC 9074
Dallas, TX 75235
Ph. 214-648-2609
Fax: 214-648-2086

United Blood Services
2325 Pershing Dr.
P.O. Box 3547
El Paso, TX 79923
http://aztec.asu.edu/blood

United Blood Services
1312 Pecan Blvd.
McAllen, TX 78501
Ph. 210-682-1314
Fax: 210-682-7578
http://aztec.asu.edu/blood

United Blood Services
224 E. Harris Ave.
P.O. Box 3206
San Angelo, TX 76902
Ph. 915-653-1308
Fax: 915-658-3537
http://aztec.asu.edu/blood

Utah

Intermountain Organ Recovery System
230 S. 500 East, Suite 290
Salt Lake City, UT 84102
Ph. 801-521-1755
Fax: 801-364-8815

Intermountain Tissue Center
University of Utah Medical Center
50 N. Medical Dr.
Salt Lake City, UT 84132
Ph. 801-581-4299
Fax: 801-581-3271

Utah Lions Eye Bank
John A. Moran Eye Center
University of Utah Health Science Center
75 N. Medical Dr.
Salt Lake City, UT 84132
http://insight.med.utah.edu/lions/index.html

Virginia

LifeNet Transplant Services
5809 Ward Court
Virginia Beach, VA 23455
Ph. 800-847-7831
Fax: 757-464-5721

Lions Medical Eye Bank and Research
Center of Eastern Virginia, Inc.
600 Gresham Dr.
Norfolk, VA 23507
Ph. 757-688-3937
Fax: 757-688-3744

Old Dominion Eye Bank
1001 E. Marshall St.
Richmond, VA 23219
Ph. 800-832-0728
Fax: 804-649-2879
http://www.odeb.org/default.htm

Southeast Organ Procurement Foundation
5004 Monument Ave., Suite 101
Richmond, VA 23230
Ph. 804-342-1414

Virginia Blood Services/ASTRAEA
5002 Airport Rd.
Roanoke, VA 24012
Ph. 804-563-0300
Fax: 804-563-8071

Virginia Blood Services/ASTRAEA
2201 Westwood Ave.
Richmond, VA 23230
Ph. 804-359-5100
Fax: 804-359-5379

Virginia Blood Services/ASTRAEA
853 W. Milan St.
Charlottesville, VA 22903
Ph. 804-977-8956
Fax: 804-979-4860

Virginia's OPA
1527 Huguenot Rd.
Midlothian, VA 23113
Ph. 804-794-4122
Fax: 703-641-0211

Washington Regional Transplant Consortium
8110 Gatehouse Rd., Suite 101W
Falls Church, VA 22042
Ph. 703-641-0100
http://www.wrtc.org

Washington

Cascade Regional Blood Services
220 S. I St.
P.O. Box 2118
Tacoma, WA 98401
Ph. 253-383-2553
Fax: 253-572-6340

Inland Northwest Blood Center
507 S. Washington
P.O. Box 1512
Spokane, WA 99210
Ph. 509-624-0151
Fax: 509-624-5484
http://www.inbc2.org

LifeCenter Northwest
2553 76th Ave, S.E.
Mercer Island, WA 98040-2758
Ph. 888-543-3287
Fax: 206-329-5433

Northwest Tissue Center
921 Terry Ave.
Seattle, WA 98104
Ph. 206-292-1879
Fax: 206-343-5043
http://www.nwtc.org

Puget Sound Blood Center
921 Terry Ave.
Seattle, WA 98104
Ph. 800-398-7888
http://www.psbc.org

Wisconsin

Blood Center of Southeastern Wisconsin
638 N. 18th St.
P.O. Box 2178
Milwaukee, WI 53201
Ph. 414-933-5000
Fax: 414-933-6803
http://www.bloodctrwise.org

Community Blood Bank
4406 W. Spencer St.
Appleton, WI 54915
Ph. 920-738-3131
Fax: 920-738-3139

The Eyebank of Wisconsin, Inc.
2870 University Ave., Suite 103
Madison, WI 53705-3611
Ph. 877-233-2354
Fax: 608-233-2895
http://www.eyebankwis.com/

Marathon County Blood Bank
404 S. Third Ave.
Wausau, WI 54401
Ph. 715-842-0761
Fax: 715-845-6429

University of Wisconsin OPO
600 Highland Ave.
Madison, WI 53792
Ph. 608-263-1341
Fax: 608-262-9099

Wisconsin Donor Network
9200 W. Wisconsin Ave.
Milwaukee, WI 53226
Ph. 414-259-2024
Fax: 206-259-8059

Wyoming

United Blood Services
2021 Warren Ave.
P.O. Box 1248
Cheyenne, WY 82003
Ph. 307-638-3326
Fax: 307-638-1932
http://aztec.asu.edu/blood

CRYOPRESERVATION STORAGE FACILITIES AND FERTILITY CLINICS BY STATE

The following is a partial list of cryopreservation storage facilities and fertility clinics (with egg, sperm, and embryo storage facilities) in the United States.

Arizona	Arizona Reproductive Medicine and Gynecology, Ltd. 2850 N. 24th St., Suite 503 Phoenix, AZ 85008 Ph. 602-468-3840 Fax: 602-468-2449 http://www.conceive.com
	IVF Phoenix 4626 E. Shea Blvd. Building C, Suite C-230 Phoenix, AZ 85028 Ph. 602-996-2411 Fax: 602-996-5254 http://www.ihr.com/ivfphoenix/index.html
	West Valley Fertility Center 6525 West Sack Dr., Suite 208 Glendale, AZ 85308 Ph. 623-561-8636 Fax: 623-561-2522 http://www.wvfc.com
California	Alta Bates In Vitro Fertilization Program Stanford University Medical Ctr. 2999 Regent St. #101A Berkeley, CA 94705 Ph. 510-649-0440 Fax: 510-649-8700
	California Cryobank 1019 Gayley Ave. Los Angeles, CA 90024 Ph. 310-443-5244 Fax: 310-443-5258

California Cryobank
770 Welch Rd., Suite 170
Palo Alto, CA 94304
Ph. 650-324-1900
Fax: 650-324-1946

California North Bay Fertility Association
1111 Sonoma Ave., Suite 214
Santa Rosa, CA 65405
Ph. 707-575-5831
Fax: 707-575-4379
http://www.ihr.com/cnbfa/

The Fertility Institutes
18370 Burbank Blvd., Suite 414
Tarzana, CA 91356
Ph. 818-776-8700
Fax: 818-776-8700
http://www.fertility-docs.com

IGO Medical Group of San Diego
9339 Genesee Ave., Suite 220
San Diego, CA 94305
Ph. 619-455-7520
Fax: 619-554-1312
http://www.ihr.com/igo/

Northern California Fertility Center
406 1/2 Sunrise Ave.
Suite 3A
Roseville, CA 95661
Ph. 916-773-2229
Fax: 916-773-8391
http://www.ncfmc.com

NOVA In Vitro Fertilization Clinic
1681 El Camino Real
Palo Alto, CA 94306
Ph. 650-322-0500
Fax: 650-322-5404
http://www.novaivf.com

Reproductive Endocrinology and Infertility Program
Stanford Univ. Medical Ctr.
300 Pasteur Dr.
Stanford University
Stanford, CA 94305
Ph. 650-725-5983
http://www.stanford.edu/dept/GYNOB/rei

The Sperm Bank of California
Reproductive Technologies, Inc.
2115 Milvia St., 2nd Floor
Berkeley, CA 94704
Ph. 510-841-1858
Fax: 510-841-0332
http://www.thespermbankofca.org

UCSF IVF Program
350 Parnassus Ave.
Suite 300
San Francisco, CA 94117
Ph. 415-476-2224
Fax: 415-476-1811
http://www.ihr.com/ussfivf/index.html

West Coast Infertility Medical Center, Inc.
250 N. Robertson Blvd., Suite 403
Beverly Hills, CA 90211
Ph. 310-285-0333
Fax: 310-285-0334

Zygen Laboratories
18425 Burbank Blvd., Suite #411
Tarzana, CA 91356
Ph. 800-255-7242
Fax: 818-705-3640

Colorado

CryoGam Colorado, Inc.
1805 E. 18th St.
Loveland, CO 80538
Ph. 800-473-9601
http://www.cryogam.com

Florida

Center for Advanced Reproductive Endocrinology
6738 W. Sunrise Blvd.
Suite 106
Plantation, FL 33313
Ph. 954-584-2273
Fax: 954-587-9660
http://www.care-life.com/

Cryobanks International, Inc.
270 S. Northlake Blvd., #1012
Altamonte Springs, FL 32701
Ph. 407-834-8333
Fax: 407-834-3533
http://www.uscryo-cord.com/index.html

The Repository
Sperm and Embryo Bank
1930 N.E. 47th Street, Suite 105
Ft. Lauderdale, FL 33308
Ph. 954-351-7030
Fax: 954-351-9060
http://www.safari.net/~sperm/index.html

Georgia

Xytex
1100 Emmett St.
Augusta, GA 30904
Ph. 706-733-0130
Fax: 706-736-9720

Illinois

Advanced Fertility Center of Chicago
6440 Grand Ave., Suite 102
Gurnee, IL 60031
Ph. 847-855-1818
http://www.advancedfertility.com

Reproductive Genetics Institute
836 W. Wellington Ave.
Chicago, IL 60657
Ph. 773-296-7095
Fax: 773-871-5221
http://www.globexnet.com/rgi/rgi7.htm

Iowa

The Iowa Women's Health Center
Advanced Reproductive Care
2 Boyd Tower
The University of Iowa Hospitals and Clinics
200 Hawkins Dr.
Iowa City, IA 52242
Ph. 319-356-8483
Fax: 319-353-6659
http://www.uihc.uiowa.edu/arc

Kansas

Reproductive Resource Ctr. of Greater Kansas City
12200 W. 106th, Suite 120
Overland Park, KS 66215
Ph. 913-894-2323
Fax: 913-894-0841
http://www.rrcgkc.com

Maryland

Fertility Center of Maryland
110 West Rd., Suite 102
Towson, MD 21204
Ph. 410-296-6400
Fax: 410-296-6405
http://www.erols.com/fcmivf/index.html

GBMC—Fertility Center
6569 N. Charles St.
Physicians Pavilion West
Suite 406
Baltimore, MD 21204
Ph. 410-828-3109
Fax: 410-828-3067
http://www.gbmc.org/services/fertility_center

Shady Grove Fertility Center
15001 Shady Grove Rd.
Suite 400
Rockville, MD 20850
Ph. 301-340-1188
Fax: 301-340-1612
http://www2.shadygrovefertility.com/sgfc

Massachusetts

California Cryobank, Inc.
955 Massachusetts Ave.
Cambridge, MA 02139
Ph. 617-497-8646
Fax: 617-497-6531

Fertility Ctr. of New England, Inc.
20 Pond Meadow Dr.
Suite 101
Reading, MA 01867
Ph. 781-942-7000
Fax: 781-942-7200
http://www.fertilitycenter.com

Reproductive Science Center of Boston
Deaconess Waltham Hospital
Hope Ave.
Waltham, MA 02254
Ph. 617-647-6263
Fax: 617-647-6323
http://www.cris.com/~rscboston/

Minnesota

Cryogenic Laboratories, Inc.
1944 Lexington Ave. N.
Roseville, MN 55113
Ph. 800-466-2796
Fax: 651-489-8989
http://www.cryolab.com

Montana

Northwest Andrology & Cryobank, Inc.
2825 Fort Missoula Rd.
Physicians Center #1, Suite 121
Missoula, MT 59804
Ph. 406-549-0958
http://www.nwcryobank.com

New Jersey

Sperm & Embryo Bank of New Jersey
1130 Rte. 22W, P.O. Box 1290
Mountainside, NJ 07092
Ph. 800-637-7776
Fax: 908-232-2114

North Carolina

North Carolina Center for Reproductive Medicine
400 Ashville Ave., Suite 200
Cary, NC 27511
Ph. 919-233-1680
Fax: 919-233-1685
http://www.nccrm.com/nccrm/

Ohio

Andrology Laboratory & Sperm Bank
The Cleveland Clinic Foundation
9500 Euclid Ave., Desk A19.1
Cleveland, OH 44195
Ph. 800-223-2273, ext. 48182
Fax: 216-445-6049

Cryobiology, Inc.
4830D Knightsville Blvd.
Columbus, OH 43214
Ph. 614-451-4375
Fax: 614-451-5284

Genetics and IVF Institute of Ohio
369 W. First Street, Suite 120
Dayton, OH 45402
Ph. 937-418-GIVF
http://www.erienet.com/givf

Oregon

OHSU Fertility Consultants
1750 S.W. Harbor Way, Suite 100
Portland, OR 97201
Ph. 503-418-3750
Fax: 503-418-3767
http://www.ihr.com/oregon/

Pennsylvania

Fertility Center
Geisinger Medical Center
Danville, PA 17821
Ph. 570-271-5620
Fax: 570-271-5629
http://www.hslc.org/~rshabanowitz/index.htm

Reproductive Science Institute
950 West Valley Rd.
Suite 2401
Wayne, PA 19087
Ph. 610-964-9663
Fax: 610-964-0536

Women's Institute for Fertility, Endocrinology, and Menopause
815 Locust St.
Philadelphia, PA 19107
Ph. 215-922-2206
Fax: 215-922-3777
http://www.womensinstitute.org

Tennessee

The Center for Applied Reproductive Science
Johnson City Medical Ctr. Office Bldg
408 State of Franklin Rd.
Johnson City, TN 37604
Ph. 423-461-8880
Fax: 423-461-8887
http://www.ivf-et.com

The Center for Reproductive Health
326 21st Ave. N.
Nashville, TN 37203
Ph. 615-321-8899
Fax: 615-321-8877
http://www.reproductivehealthctr.com/

Texas

Fertility Center of San Antonio
4499 Medical Dr., Suite 360
San Antonio, TX 78229
Ph. 210-692-0577
Fax: 210-692-1210
http://www.fertilityusa.com

North Houston Center for Reproductive Medicine
530 Wells Fargo Dr., Suite 116
Houston, TX 77090
Ph. 281-444-4784
Fax: 281-444-0429
http://www.ihr.com/nhcrm/

Virginia

Dominion Fertility and Endocrinology
46 S. Glebe Rd., Suite 301
Arlington, VA 22204
Ph. 703-920-3890
Fax: 703-892-6037
http://www2.dominionfertility.com/df/

Genetics and IVF Institute
Fairfax Cryobank
3015 Williams Dr., #110
Fairfax, VA 22301
Ph. 800-338-8407
Fax: 703-698-3933
http://www.givf.com
http://fairfaxcryobank.com

Jones Institute for Reproductive Medicine
601 Colley Ave.
Norfolk, VA 23507
Ph. 757-446-7100

STORED TISSUE SAMPLE WEB SITES

Advanced Fertility Center of Chicago	http://www.advancedfertility.com
Alabama Community Blood Bank	http://www.crbs.org
Alabama Eye Bank	http://www.uab.edu/eye/eyebank3.html
Alabama Organ Center	http://www.uab.edu/aoc/
Alzheimer Center—Case Western Reserve University	http://www.ohioalzcenter.org
Alzheimer's Disease Center— Northwestern University	http://www.brain.nwu.edu/core/index.htm
Alzheimer's Disease Center— University of Kansas Medical Center	http://www.kumc.edu/instruction/medicine/neurology/ resAD.htm
Alzheimer's Disease Center— University of California, Davis	http://alzheimer.ucdavis.edu/adc
Alzheimer's Disease Core Center	http://www.visn1.org/alzheimer/BrainBank.htm
Alzheimer's Disease Research Center—Baylor College of Medicine	http://www.bcm.tmc.edu/neurol struct/adrc/adrc1.html
Alzheimer's Disease Research Center—University of Southern California	http://www.usc.edu/dept/gero/ADRC
Alzheimer's Disease Research Center—Washington University	http://www.adrc.wustl.edu/adrc/adrc2.html
American Association of Tissue Banks	http://www.aatb.org/aatbac.htm
American Red Cross	http:// www.redcross.org
Arizona Reproductive Medicine and Gynecology, Ltd.	http://www.conceive.com
Armed Forces DNA Laboratory	http://www.afip.org/homes/oafme/dna/afdil.html
Atlanta LifeSouth Community Blood Centers	http://www.crbs.org
Blood Assurance, Inc.	http://www.bloodassurance.org
Blood and Tissue Center of Central Texas	http://www.austin.citysearch.com/E/V/AUSTX/0004/52/ 93/11.html
Blood Bank of Alaska, Inc.	http://www.customcpu.com/np/bba/default.htm
Blood Bank of the Redwoods	http:/bbr.org
Blood Center for Southeast Louisiana	http://www.thebloodcenter.org
Blood Center of Central Iowa	http://www.bloodonor.org
Blood Center of New Jersey	http://www.bloodnj.org

Blood Center of Southeastern Wisconsin	http://www.bloodctrwise.org
Blood Centers of the Pacific	http://www.citysearch.com/sfo/bloodcenter
Brain and Tissues Bank for Developmental Disorders— Children's Hospital of Orange County	http://www.choc.com/btbmain.htm
Brain and Tissues Bank for Developmental Disorders— University of Maryland	http://www.som1.umaryland.edu/BTBank
Brain and Tissues Bank for Developmental Disorders— University of Miami	http://www.med.miami.edu/BTB
Brain Bank—Medical College of Georgia	http://www.mcg.edu/Centers/Alz/arc.htm
CALGB Central Office	http://128.135.31.4
California Cancer Registry	http://www.ccrcal.org
California North Bay Fertility Association	http://www.ihr.com/cnbfa/
California Tumor Registry	http://www.llu.edu/llu.cttr
Cancer Data Registry of Idaho	http://www.idcancer.org
Center for Advanced Reproductive Endocrinology	http://www.care-life.com/
Centers for Disease Control and Prevention (CDC)	http://www.cdc.gov/
Central California Blood Center	http://www.cencalblood.org/default02.htm
Central Florida Lions Eye and Tissue Bank, Inc.	http://www.lionseyebank.com/home.html
Central Illinois Community Blood Bank	http://www.fgi.net/~bloodbnk
Central Indiana Regional Blood Center Tissue Bank	http://www.donor-link.org
Central Maine Medical Center	http://www2.cmmc.org/cmmc/cancercare/registry.html
Central New Jersey Blood Center	http://www.cjbc.org
Colorado Central Cancer Registry	http://sedac.ciesin.org/ozone/regs/colorado.html
Community Blood Bank of Erie County	http://www.eriebloodbank.org
Community Blood Center of Greater Kansas City	http://kcblood.org
Cord Blood Registry	http://www.cordblood.com
Coriell Institute for Medical Research	http://arginine.umdnj.edu/info.html
CryoBanks International, Inc.	http://www.uscryo-cord.com/index.html
CryoGam Colorado, Inc.	http://www.cryogam.com
Cryogenics Laboratories, Inc.	http://www.cryolab.com
Dominion Fertility and Endocrinology	http://www2.dominionfertility.com/df/
Donor Network of Arizona	http://www.donor-network.org
East Tennessee Lions Eye Bank	http://www.korrnet.org/eyebank/index.html
Emory University's Alzheimer's Disease Center	http://www.emory.edu/WHSC/MED/ADC

Fairfax Cryobank	http://fairfaxcryobank.com
Federal Bureau of Investigations (FBI)	http://www.fbi.gov/
Fertility Center—Geisinger Medical Center	http://www.hslc.org/~rshabanowitz/index.htm
Fertility Center of Maryland	http://www.erols.com/fcmivf/index.html
Fertility Center of New England, Inc.	http://www.fertilitycenter.com
Fertility Center of San Antonio	http://www.fertilityusa.com
Florida Blood Services	http://www.fbsblood.org
Florida Cancer Data System	http://fdcs.med.miami.edu/
Florida Georgia Blood Alliance	http://www.fgba.org
Forensic Science Research and Training Center	http://www.fbi.gov/lab/report/research.htm
Genetics and IVF Institute	http://www.givf.com
Genetics and IVF Institute of Ohio	http://www.erienet.com/givf
Georgia Comprehensive Cancer Registry	http://www.ph.dhr.state.ga.us/org/cancercontrolsection.cancerregistry.htm
GOG Tissue Bank	http://www.gog.org
Great Plains Eye Bank, Inc.	http://www.ttuhsc.edu/eye/defaultpage/main/EyeBank.htm
Greater Baltimore Medical Center— Fertility Center	http://www.gbmc.org/services/fertility_center
Gulf Coast Regional Blood Center	http://www.giveblood.org
Hartford Hospital Cancer Registry	http://www.harthosp.org/cancer/registry
Harvard Brain Tissue Resource Center	http://www.mcleanhospital.org/brainbank.html
Hawaii Lions Eye Bank	http://www.eyebank.org
Hawaii Tumor Registry	http://www.planet-hawaii.com/htr
Hollings Cancer Center—High Risk Lung Cancer Registry	http://hcc.musc.edu/lungreg
Hoxworth Blood Center—University of Cincinnati Medical Center	http://www.hoxworth.org
IGO Medical Group of San Diego	http://www.ihr.com/igo
Illinois State Cancer Registry	http://hometown.aol.com/epistudies/cancer/index/htm
Indiana Alzheimer Disease Center National Cell Repository	http://medgen.iupui.edu/research/alzheimer
Inland Northwest Blood Center	http://www.inbc2.org
International Pediatric Adrenocortical Tumor Registry	http://www.stjude.org/ipactr/objectives.htm
IVF Phoenix	http://www.ihr.com/ivfphoenix/index.html
Kansas Cancer Registry	http://www.kumc.edu/som/kcr
Kathleen Price Bryan Brain Bank	http://www.medicine.mc.duke.edu/ADRC/INDEX.html
Kentucky Lions Eye Bank	http://athena.louisville.edu/medschool/ophthalmology/kleb.htm
Kentucky Cancer Registry	http://www.kcr.uky.edu
Lane Memorial Blood Bank	http://www.lanecountyblood.org
Lifeblood/Mid-South Regional Blood Center	http://www.lifeblood.com
LifeSouth Community Blood Centers	http://www.crbs.org
LifeSpan BioSciences, Inc.	http://www.lsbio.com

Lions Eye Bank of Central Texas	http://www.io.com/~garycox/LEBCT.html
Lions Eye Bank of Northwest Pennsylvania	http://www.unitedwayerie.org/eyebank
Lions Eye Bank of Oregon	http://www.orlions.org/cover.htm
Longitudinal Studies Branch of the National Institute on Aging (NIA)	http://www.grc.nia.nih.gov/Branches/lsb/lsb.htm
Massachusetts General Hospital Cancer Data Registry	http://cancer.mgh.harvard.edu/tumreg/tumreg.htm
Massachusetts General Hospital Tumor Bank	http://cancer.mgh.harvard.edu/tumorbank
Medical Eye Bank of Florida	http://www.castlegate.net/MEBFL/index.htm
Memorial Blood Centers of Minnesota	http://www.mbcm.org
Metropolitan New York Registry	http://www.med.nyu.edu/Biostat-Epi/mnyr.htm
Michigan Alzheimer's Disease Research Center	http://www.med.umich.edu/madrc/MADRC.html
Michigan Community Blood Centers	http://miblood.org
Michigan Eye Bank	http://www.mebtc.org
Missouri Lions Eye Research Foundation	http://www.rollanet.org/~rlions/mlerf
Mucosal Immunology Core—UCLA	http://www.medsch.ucla.edu/aidsinst/cfar/Mucosal.htm
National Cancer Institute (NCI)	http://www.nci.nih.gov
National Center for Environmental Health (NCEH)	http://www.cdc.gov/nceh/ncehhome.htm
National Center for Infectious Diseases (NCID)	http://www.cdc.gov/ncidod/ncid.htm
National Disease Research Interchange	http://www.ndri.com
National Familial Lung Cancer Registry	http://www.path.jhu.edu/nfltr.html
National Health and Nutrition Examination Survey (NHANES)	http://www.cdc.gov/ncnswww/about/major/nhanes/nhanes.htm
National Heart, Lung, and Blood Institute (NHLBI)	http://www.nhlbi.nih.gov/nhlbi/nhlbi.htm
National Institute of Environmental Health Sciences	http://www.niehs.nih.gov
National Institute of Allergy and Infectious Disease (NIAID)	http://www.niaid.nih.gov/
National Institutes of Health (NIH)	http://www.nih.gov/index.html
National Institute of Mental Health (NIMH)	http://www.nimh.nih.gov/
National Institute on Aging	http://www.nih.gov/nia
National NeuroAIDS Tissue Consortium	http://www.nimh.nih.gov/oa/nntnhome.htm
National Neurological Research Specimen Bank	http://loni.ucla.edu/~nnrsb/nnrsb
National Pathology Repository	http://www.afip.mil/repository/welcome.html
National Psoriasis Tissue Bank	http://www.psoriasis.org/tissuebank.html

National Temporal Bone, Hearing, and Balance Pathology Resource Registry	http://www.tbregistry.org
National Wilms Tumor Study Group	http://www.nwtsg.org
NCI AIDS Malignancy Bank	http://cancernet.nci.nih.gov/amb/amb.html
NCI Breast Cancer Specimen and Data Information System	http://www.napbc.ims.nci.nih.gov/
NCI Cooperative Breast Cancer Tissue Resource (CBCTR)	http://www-cbctr.ims.nci.nih.gov
NCI Cooperative Family Registry for Breast Cancer Studies (CFRBCS)	http://www-dceg.ims.nci.nih.gov/cfrbcs
NCI Cooperative Human Tissue Network (CHTN)	http://www-chtn.ims.nci.nih.gov/
NCI Clinical Trials Cooperative Group	http://www.specimens.ims.nci.nih.gov/about.html
NCI Surveillance, Epidemiology, and End Results Program	http://www-seer.ims.nci.nih.gov
New England Cord Blood Bank	http://www.cordbloodbank.com/overview.htm
New England Organ Bank	http://www.neob.org
New Jersey Organ and Tissue Sharing Network	http://www.sharenj.org
New Jersey State Cancer Registry	http://www.ker.state.nj.us/health/cancer/njscr1b.htm
New York Blood Center	http://www.nybloodcenter.org
NIH Women's Health Initiative (WHI)	http://odp.ld.nih.gov/whi/
North Carolina Cancer Registry	http://www.schs.state.nc.us/SCHS/about/branches/ccr.html
North Carolina Center for Reproductive Medicine	http://www.nccrm.com/nccrm/
North Houston Center for Reproductive Medicine	http://www.ihr.com/nhcrm
Northern Californa Fertility Center	http://www.ncfmc.com
Northwest Andrology and Cryobank, Inc.	http://www.nwcryobank.com
Northwest Tissue Center	http://www.nwtc.org
NOVA In Vitro Fertilization Clinic	http://www.novaivf.com
Old Dominion Eye Bank	http://www.odeb.org/default.htm
Oklahoma Lions Eye Bank	http://www.ionet.net/~oleb/lionseye.html
Oregon Health Sciences University Fertility Consultants	http://www.ihr.com/oregon
Oregon State Cancer Registry	http://www.orcpr.org/oscar.html
PathServe Autopsy and Tissue Bank	http://www.tissuebank.com
POG Operations Office	http://www.pog.ufl.edu
Puget Sound Blood Center	http://www.psbc.org
Regional Organ Bank of Illinois	http://www.robi.org
Reproductive Endocrinology and Infertility Program	http://www.stanford.edu/dept/GYNOB/rei
Reproductive Genetics Institute	http://www.globexnet.com/rgi/rgi7.htm
Reproductive Resource Center of Greater Kansas City	http://www.rrcgkc.com

Reproductive Science Center of Boston	http://www.cris.com/~rscboston/
Resource for Tumor Tissue and Data—NYU School of Medicine	http://kccc-www.med.nyu.edu/RTTD.htm
Rhode Island Blood Center	http://www.ribc.org
Rhode Island Cancer Registry	http://www.health.state.ri.us/canrep.htm
Rochester Eye and Human Parts Bank	http://www.rehpb.org
Rocky Mountain Lions Eye Bank	http://www.corneas.org
Rocky Mountain Multiple Sclerosis Center Tissue Bank	http://www.swedmc.com:80/msc/tissue.htm
Rush Alzheimer's Disease Center (Rush Brain Bank)	http://www.rush.edu/Departments/Alzheimers/Research.html
San Diego Blood Bank	http://www.sandiegobloodbank.org
Sarasota Community Blood Bank	http://www.sarasota-online.com/scbb
Savannah River Region Cancer Incidence Registry	http://www.musc.edu/srrhis/
Shady Grove Fertility Center	http://www2.shadygrovefertility.com/sgfc
Shepeard Community Blood Center	http://www.shepeardblood.com
South Carolina OPA	http://www.midnet.sc.edu/scopa/scopa.htm
South Georgia Branch of Southeastern Community Blood Center	http://www.scbcinfo.org
South Texas Blood and Tissue Center	http://www.bloodntissue.org
Southeastern Community Blood Center	http://www.scbcinfo.org
Southwest Organ Bank	http://wg.dzn.com/swob/top.htm
Southwest Transplant Alliance	http://www.organ.org
St. Louis Cord Blood Bank	http://www.slu.edu/colleges/med/departments/pediatrics/cordbank/moreinfo.html
State Health Registry of Iowa	http://www.uiowa.edu/~vpr/research/organize/healthreg.htm
Taub Center for Alzheimer's Disease Research—Columbia University	http://pathology.cpmc.columbia.edu/ADNP.html
Tennessee Donor Services	http://www.korrnet.org/donors
Texas Cancer Data Center	http://www.txcancer.org
The Center for Applied Reproductive Science	http://www.ivf-et.com
The Center for Reproductive Health	http://www.reproductivehealthctr.com/
The Eyebank of Wisconsin, Inc.	http://www.eyebankwis.com
The Fertility Institutes	http://www.fertility-docs.com
The Iowa Women's Health Center Advanced Reproductive Care	http://www.uihc.uiowa.edu/arc
The Repository Sperm and Embryo Bank	http://www.safari.net/~sperm/index.html
The Sperm Bank of California	http://www.thespermbankofca.org
United Blood Services	http://aztec.asu.edu/blood
University of California, San Francisco, IVF Program	http://www.ihr.com/ucsfivf/index.html
University of California, San Francisco, Cancer Center Tissue Core	http://cc.ucsf.edu/tissue/index.html

Utah Lions Eye Bank	http://www.insight.med.utah.edu/lions/index.html
Vermont Cancer Registry	http://www.senate.gov/~leahy/bcreg.htm
Virginia Cancer Registry	http://www.vdh.state.va.us/epi/ver.htm
Washington Regional Transplant Consortium	http://www.wrtc.org
Washington State Cancer Registry	http://www.doh.wa.gov/ehspl/epidemiology/wscr1.htm
West Valley Fertility Center	http://www.wvfc.com
Wichita Eye Bank	http://www2.southwind.net/~gsbryan
Wisconsin Cancer Reporting System	http://www.dhfs.state.wi.us/wcrs/object.htm
Women's Institute for Fertility, Endocrinology, and Menopause	http://www.womensinstitute.org
Wyoming Cancer Surveillance	http://wdhfs.state.wy.us/cancer

American Medical Association, *Graduate Medical Education Directory 1997-1998,* Chicago: American Medical Association, 1997.

Andrews, L. B., *State Laws and Regulations Governing Newborn Screening,* Chicago: American Bar Foundation, 1995.

Bailar, J. C., III, "Monitoring Human Tissues for Toxic Substances: A Follow-Up to the National Academy of Sciences (NAS) Report," *Environmental Health Perspectives,* 103 (supplement 3), 1995, pp. 81–84.

Clinical Laboratory Improvement Amendments, Clinical Laboratory Improvement Amendments of 1988 (CLIA), 42 CFR 493 (10-1-96 Edition), 1996, pp. 796–921.

Department of Health and Human Services, Clinical Laboratory Improvement Amendments (CLIA), November 29, 1991, Press Release 1991.11.29.

Eye Bank Association of America, "1997 Eyebanking Statistics Report," accessed at http://www.restoresight.org, 1998.

Finn, P., "Revolution Underway in Use of DNA Profiles. Bid to Link U.S. Databanks Is Crime-Solving Edge," *Washington Post,* November 16, 1997, p. B4.

Gluckman, E., H. E. Broxmeyer, A. D. Auerbach, et al., "Hematopoietic Reconstitution in a Patient with Fanconi's Anemia by Means of Umbilical-Cord Blood from an HLA-Identical Sibling," *New England Journal of Medicine,* 321, 1989, pp. 1174–1178.

Graduate Medical Education, *Journal of the American Medical Association,* 278(9), 1997, Appendix II, pp. 775–784.

Graeber, M. B., S. Kösel, R. Egensperger, R. B. Banati, U. Müller, K. Bise, P. Hoff, H. J. Möller, K. Fujisawa, and P. Mehraein, "Rediscovery of the Case Described by Alois Alzheimer in 1911: Historical, Histological, and Molecular Genetic Analysis," *Neurogenetics,* 1(1), 1997 p. 73–80.

Graeber, M. B., S. Kösel, E. Grabson-Frodl, H. J. Möller, and P. Mehraein, "Histopathology and APOE Genotype of the First Alzheimer Disease Patient, Auguste D.," *Neurogenetics,* 1(3), 1998, pp. 223–228.

Holmes, M., "Man Cleared of Rape to Be Pardoned," Associated Press, October 8, 1997.

McEwen, J. E., "DNA Data Banks," in M. A. Rothstein, ed., *Genetic Secrets: Protecting Privacy and Confidentiality in the Genetic Era,* New Haven, Conn.: Yale University Press, 1997, Chapter 11.

McEwen, J. E., and P. R. Reilly, "Stored Guthrie Cards as DNA 'Banks,'" *American Journal of Human Genetics,* 55, 1994, pp. 196–200.

McEwen, J. E., and P. R. Reilly, "A Survey of DNA Diagnostic Laboratories Regarding DNA Banking," *American Journal of Human Genetics,* 56(6), 1995, pp. 1477–1486.

Mertz, J. F., P. Sanker, S. E. Taube, and V. Livoisi, "Use of Human Tissues in Research: Clarifying Clinician and Researcher Roles and Information Flows," *Journal of Investigative Medicine,* 45(5), 1997, pp. 252–257.

National Bioethics Advisory Commission, "Research Involving Human Biological Materials: Ethical Issues and Policy Guidance, Volume 1," accessed at http://bioethics.gov/cgi-bin/bioeth_counter.pl, 1999.

National Heart, Lung, and Blood Institute, "Blood Specimen Repository: 1996 Catalog," 1996.

Perdahl-Wallace, E. B., "Placental Cord Blood Transplantation," *Transplant Forum,* 4(2), 1997, pp. 4–5.

Reilly, P., "ASHG Statement on Genetics and Privacy: Testimony to U.S. Congress," *American Journal of Human Genetics,* 50, 1992, pp. 640–642.

Sugarman, J., V. Kaalund, E. Kodish, M. F. Marshall, E. G. Reisner, B. S. Wilfond, and P. R. Wolpe, "Ethical Issues in Umbilical Cord Blood Banking," *Journal of the American Medical Association,* 278(11), 1997, pp. 938–943.

Technical Working Group on DNA Analysis Methods (TWGDAM), "The Combined DNA Index System (CODIS): A Theoretical Model," in L. T. Kirby, ed., *DNA Fingerprinting: An Introduction,* New York: Stockton Press, 1989, pp. 279–317.

Torloni, A. S., "Umbilical Cord Cells: A Viable Alternative for BMT," *Transplant Forum,* 4(2), 1997, p. 6.

Wagner, J. E., N. A. Kernan, M. Steinbuch, H. E. Broxmeyer, and E. Gluckman, "Allogeneic Sibling Umbilical Cord Blood Transplantation in Children with Malignant and Nonmalignant Disease," *Lancet,* 346, 1995, pp. 214–219.

Wagner, J. E., J. Rosenthal, R. Sweetman, et al., "Successful Transplantation of HLA-Matched and HLA-Mismatched Umbilical Cord Blood from Unrelated Donors: Analysis of Engraftment and Acute Graft-Versus-Host Disease," *Blood,* 88, 1996, pp. 795–802.

Wise, S. A., and B. J. Koster, "Considerations in the Design of an Environmental Specimen Bank: Experiences of the National Biomonitoring Specimen Bank Program," *Environmental Health Perspectives,* 103 (supplement 3), 1995, pp. 61–67.